DIZZINESS:
A Guide to Disorders of Balance

TONY WRIGHT DM, FRCS (Ed), TechRMS

Senior Lecturer in Otology,
The Institute of Laryngology and Otology,
London

CROOM HELM
London & Sydney

© 1988 Tony Wright
Croom Helm Ltd, Provident House, Burrell Row,
Beckenham, Kent BR3 1AT
Croom Helm Australia, 44-50 Waterloo Road,
North Ryde, 2113, New South Wales

British Library Cataloguing in Publication Data

Wright, Tony
    Dizziness: a guide to disorders of
    balance.
    1. Vertigo
    I. Title
    616.8′41   RB150.V4

    ISBN 0-7099-3659-1

Distributed exclusively in the USA by Sheridan House Inc.,
145 Palisade Street, Dobbs Ferry NY 10522

Typeset by Leaper & Gard Ltd, Bristol, England
Printed and bound in Great Britain by
Biddles Ltd, Guildford and King's Lynn

Contents

Acknowledgements

The writing of this book has been made possible by those who taught me both directly and by way of their publications. It is impossible to acknowledge the contributor of each idea or turn of phrase that best expresses a clinical situation or dilemma and so I hope that this generalised expression of my gratitude is adequate.

The patience of Job has been shown both by Tim Hardwick, senior editor at Croom Helm, in waiting for the text and by Linda Steele in persevering and producing the final type written copy. The Department of Medical Photography of the Institute of Laryngology and Otology has been invaluable in helping produce the finished illustrations.

Gerald Duckworth and Co. are also to be thanked for allowing the use of a passage from 'The man who mistook his wife for a hat' by Oliver Sacks.

I am extremely grateful to Duphar Laboratories Limited for their help in enabling me to include colour plates in this book.

Introduction

This is not a book for experts but I hope that experts will not find too much that disappoints them or with which they disagree. Instead I have aimed it at final year medical students and junior hospital doctors, especially those preparing for examinations. But I also hope that interested general practitioners, or those preparing themselves for this exacting field, will find the book useful, as well as scientists with an interest in audiology.

Dizziness is a difficult condition, and having to diagnose and manage the dizzy patient may seem like being thrown in at the deep end when you can only just swim. The subjective nature of the complaint and the wide range of underlying problems that can cause the symptom might make you feel that you need to know something about everything before you can even hope to start understanding the condition. I have tried to rationalise making a diagnosis by describing the different types of symptom that can occur with disorder in various parts of the body so that taking the history and examining the patient follows a logical pattern. Equipment more complicated than an ophthalmoscope, auriscope and tuning fork is not really needed as a sound idea of what is going on can usually be made by taking a good history and performing a careful and thorough examination.

The more common conditions — and a few uncommon problems — are described and I have tried to indicate when and how you can manage the patient and when specialist help should be sought.

You can not hope to cure everyone who complains of dizziness, but surprisingly simple remedies often help overcome many of the problems, provided you have the enthusiasm to listen and to ask the right questions.

A. Wright
London 1987

1

Normal Balance

Dizziness in any of its many different forms is not a disease as such but the result of some underlying disorder. To make sense of the many symptoms and signs that can occur when something does go wrong it is helpful to understand how the normal system works to maintain stability. Our balance mechanisms provide us with two major functions. First, they usually prevent us from falling over and injuring ourselves, which is especially important with our intrinsically unstable two-legged way of walking . The second function they have is related to vision. The retina has maximum resolution and the best colour perception in a small region called the fovea of the macula. The position of the eyes is therefore maintained so that they continue to look at the same visual feature despite alterations in the position of the head.

To be able to perform these tasks a fairly complex arrangement has evolved with the whole network being called the vestibular system. The detailed anatomy and physiology of this is difficult with much still unknown, even to the experts. Luckily, we can dispense with virtually all of the detail as the vestibular system can very conveniently be split into its component parts and each part treated more or less separately.

An overall view of the system can also be simplified by thinking of balance as a reflex. There is a sensory input which tells the central processing unit how posture and the visual field are changing in relationship to the environment. The motor output from the central unit then acts to maintain the stability of the body and direction of gaze.

The sensory input to the system can be assigned to three major compartments as shown in Figure 1.1.

Figure 1.1: Schematic outline of the components of the vestibular system. Arrows indicate the directions of flow of sensory input and response. There are direct pathways from labyrinth and somatosensors to cerebellum but these have not been drawn in to prevent the diagram from becoming a spider's web.

THE VESTIBULAR SYSTEM

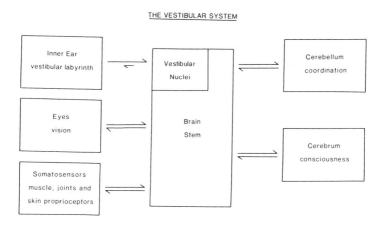

The first compartment contains the vestibular labyrinth which is located in the inner ear and which gives information about linear and angular acceleration of the head. The second contains the eyes which give information not only about movement of the head and body relative to the surroundings and vice versa, but also about what is up and what is down. This can be deduced from visual features such as the horizon, walls of buildings, the direction of rain falling in air or even of bubbles rising underwater, and experience accumulated from infancy allows us to interpret these features. The third compartment contains the sensors within the body that detect the relationship of various parts of the body to each other, and of the whole body to the outside. Touch and pressure receptors in the skin, the muscle spindles, and the joint position sensors all feed this information along the spinal cord to the brain, and are termed the somatosensors. They are particularly well developed in the muscles and joints of the neck.

Information from all three systems passes variously into the brainstem and cerebellum. Together these co-ordinate the sensory input, determine the appropriate response to alteration

3

in the incoming information, and send out the correct instructions to compensate smoothly for the changes that have occurred. These instructions are directed to the muscles that maintain body posture and eye position. The interactions within the brainstem are complex and incompletely understood and need trouble us no more except to note that one group of brainstem nuclei, the vestibular nuclei, appear to be of major importance in the integration of the sensory information.

The brainstem, of course, has a blood supply and this is derived more or less completely from the two vertebral arteries and their subsequent branches, many of which are end arteries. The brainstem and cerebellum are therefore prey not only to general disorders of the circulation and blood vessels but also to some specifically related to the course of the vertebral arteries within the cervical spine. The effects of seemingly trivial disease are often severe because of the lack of an effective collateral circulation to this part of the brain.

Because of the importance of the inner ear to the vestibular system, and the frequency with which it is affected by disease, its structure and workings will be outlined. This small section can be avoided by those eager to get on with more practical matters but the beauty and delicacy of the structures making up the vestibular labyrinth are worth at least a passing glance.

The sensory structures of the vestibular apparatus and cochlea are enclosed within a membranous labyrinth, a name which well describes its tortuous shape. It is filled with a high potassium–low sodium fluid called endolymph but is surrounded by perilymph, which resembles cerebrospinal fluid. All of this is enclosed within a system of cavities and canals in the densest portion of the petrous temporal bone — the bony labyrinth (Figure 1.2).

The vestibular portion of the labyrinth comprises three semicircular canals, set at approximately right angles to each other. They are called superior, posterior and lateral (or horizontal) and the five ends of the three canals — the superior and posterior canals joining at one end to form a common canal — open into the utricle. At one end of each canal is a dilatation called the ampulla. This contains the saddle-shaped crista which consists of the sensory cells and their nerves, and which serves to detect angular acceleration.

The utricle and another dilation in the membranous labyrinth, the saccule, each contain a flat sheet of sensory cells.

Figure 1.2: Diagram of the human labyrinth. This is the left ear with the cochlea at the front and the semicircular canals at the back. The membranous labyrinth which contains the sensory cells of hearing and balance is shown stippled, whilst the solid outline represents the surrounding bony labyrinth. There are two openings in the bony labyrinth — the oval and round windows, closed in life by the stapes and round window membrane respectively. The longest front to back dimension of the bony labyrinth is about 1.7 cm.

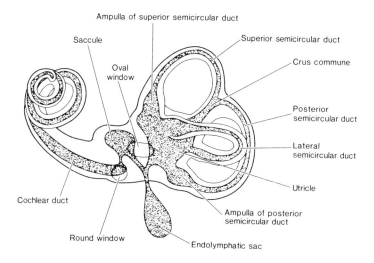

These are the maculae. They are set approximately at right angles to each other and are the detectors of linear acceleration.

Both the cristae and the maculae have the same basic structure. This is a collection of sensory cells, their supporting cells and nerves. Each sensory cell has a cluster of cilia projecting from its uppermost surface which is in contact with the endolymph. This cluster of cilia comprises a single kinocilium, which has the internal structure typical of a truly motile cilium with a 'nine plus two' arrangement of microtubules running along the length of the cilium, and numerous stereocilia. The stereocilia are poorly named as each contains a rod-like core of tightly packed actin molecules covered with a cell membrane. They are relatively rigid structures which pivot about their base when externally deflected and this action probably results in deformation of the cell body. Whatever the exact mechanism such a deflection of the stereocilia results in an alteration of the

5

resting discharge from the afferent nerve fibres that make contact with the base of the cell. If the stereocilia are deflected towards the kinocilium then the rate of discharge increases, whilst it decreases with deflection in the opposite direction (Figure 1.3).

The cells therefore have polarity dictated by the presence of the kinocilium and are found to be organised in strict patterns both within the cristae and the maculae.

Although the sensory cells are similar in these two structures the mechanism of their stimulation is different.

Figure 1.3: Simplified diagram of two vestibular sensory cells. The cell bodies are of two types. The type I cell is bottle or flask shaped and is enclosed by a nerve chalice. Type II is cylindrical and has numerous button-like nerve terminals associated with it. Projecting from the surface of each cell are many stereocilia and a single long kinocilium. At the bottom of the diagram is a representation of the firing pattern of a single nerve fibre. When the ciliary bundle is bent towards the kinocilium the nerve is stimulated and the firing rate increases. As the bundle is bent in the other direction the reverse occurs.

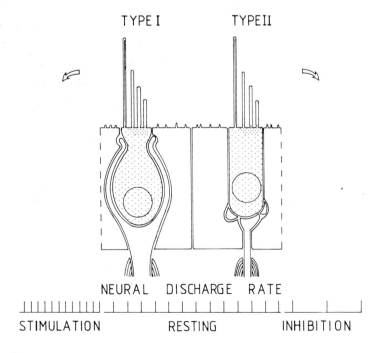

Each macula is covered by a gelatinous membrane containing many calcium carbonate crystals — the otoconia (Figure 1.4). The sensory cells are firmly attached to the underlying structures whilst the otoconial membrane lies partly in endolymph, partly on the clusters of cilia. When the head is accelerated the sensory cells move with the head but the otoconia lag behind because of their inertia. This lag is transmitted through the gelatinous membrane to cause deflection of the stereocilia and consequently the rate of firing of the afferent nerve fibres increases or decreases depending on the direction of the acceleration. When a steady speed is reached the elastic recoil of the gelatinous membrane returns the otoconial mass to its resting position and the neural output returns to its unstimulated level. When the head slows down the sensory cells slow exactly in

Figure 1.4: Diagrammatic representation of a portion of the macula. The cilia of the sensory cells are lightly embedded in a gelatinous membrane which also contains the crystals of calcium carbonate — the otoconia — on its upper surface.

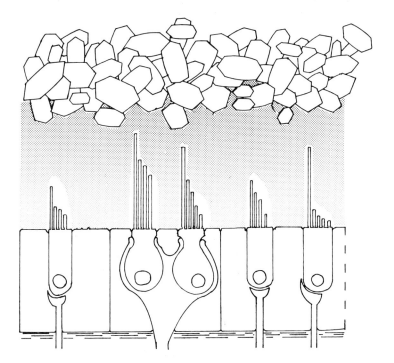

time with the head but the otoconia have momentum and continue moving so that they are slightly ahead. This relative change in position is again transmitted to the stereocilia by the gelatinous membrane but the deflection is now the opposite to that which occurred during acceleration so the change in the neural firing rate is also reversed.

The two maculae in each ear are at right angles to each other, and within each macula there are complex patterns of arrangement of the polarity of the individual cells. The lengths of the clusters of stereocilia vary from cell to cell so that overall a hugely complex pattern of signals arises during accelerations and decelerations. Figures 1.5 and 1.6 are scanning electron micrographs of the human vestibular labyrinth showing different portions of the macule of the saccule.

The mechanism of stimulation of the cells in the semicircular canals is slightly different. Instead of an otoconial membrane a gelatinous body, the cupula, sits astride the crista and in its

Figure 1.5: The surface of the macule of the saccule. The otoconial membrane has been partly removed to reveal the underlying sensory epithelium, and the tufts of the ciliary bundle can be clearly seen. Marker 10 μm.

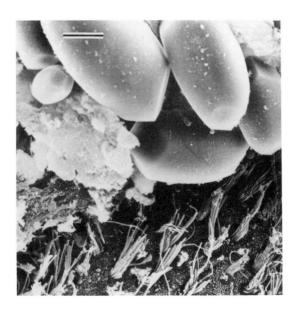

Figure 1.6: The surface of the macule of the saccule. The wide range in lengths of the ciliary clusters and the variations in the orientation of the cells can be seen at this higher magnification.

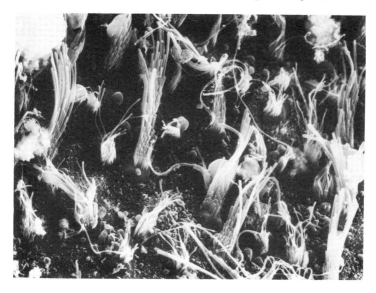

natural state extends to the walls of the ampulla. Most of the rest of the ampulla seems to be filled with a loosely packed gel. There appears to be a small gap between the cupula and the surface of the crista with the bundles of stereocilia standing in this space (Figure 1.7).

Over the years there have been many theories as to how the semicircular canals work. Most of these were based on incorrect anatomy which arose from preparation artefacts or unphysiological experiments using supra-threshold stimuli. The most likely mechanism, described by Dohlmann (1981) is that during angular acceleration of the head, the crista moves with the head as it is firmly tethered to the underlying bone by the nerves. However, the endolymph by way of its inertia tends to stay still and is therefore forced through the space between the cupula and the crista thereby deflecting the stereocilia. The angle of attachment of the semicircular canals to the ampulla and the ratio of the size of the canal to the space between the cupula and crista both serve to direct and enhance fluid movement across the surface of the crista, accounting for the extreme sensitivity of the system.

Figure 1.7: Part of the membranous labyrinth split to show the inside of the ampulla and the adjacent semicircular duct. Within the ampulla is the saddle-shaped crista (Cr) with the gelatinous cupula (Cu) astride it. Much of the dome of the ampulla is filled with a thick gelatinous meshwork indicated by the stippling. The arrow indicates the flow of endolymph across the surface of the crista. It is this flow that causes deflection of the cilia and stimulation or inhibition of the sensory cells depending on the direction of flow.

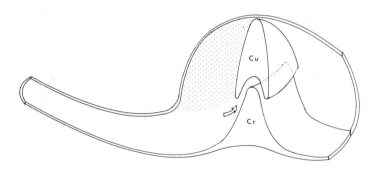

When constant rotation is reached the endolymph quickly gains momentum so that it is rotating at the same speed as the head and further stimulation does not occur as the stereocilia return to their resting position. With deceleration the endolymph carries on moving for a short while because of its recently acquired momentum and causes the reverse deflection of the stereocilia and the opposite neural output.

Since the three canals in one ear are at right angles to each other, they effectively perform a vector analysis of the applied rotation. The three canals in the other ear are complementary in position and the combined output of the six canals allows complex angular acceleration and deceleration to be analysed.

Figures 1.8 and 1.9 show the surface features of the crista from a young and an old person. There is a loss of stereocilia with ageing and this probably accounts for the loss of sensitivity of the system that is seen in old age. The term for this feature is presbyastasia.

10

Figure 1.8: The crista from the ampulla of the lateral semicircular duct of a 17 year old. The crista has curled up a little during preparation but the dense carpet of cilia can be seen on its surface. The marker is equivalent to 100 µm.

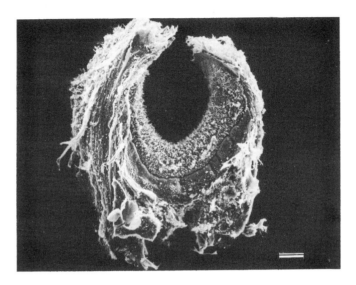

Figure 1.9: The crista, again from the ampulla of the lateral semicircular duct, but this time from a 70 year old. The ciliary carpet is missing on the crest of the crista.

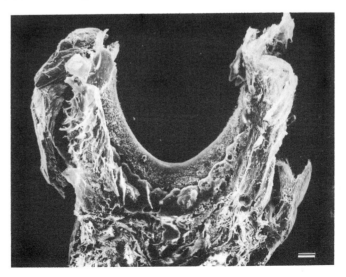

2

When Disease Strikes: The Symptoms

We are normally not aware of the smooth working of the vestibular system until something goes wrong with it when the effects can be unsettling if minimal but alarming and even dangerous when severe. A variety of sensations arise when different parts of the system are affected by disease and it is these sensations that provide the key to narrowing down the site of the disorder. It is often very difficult for 'dizzy' patients with problems to put into words their exact feelings but it is important to establish what it is they feel so that time, patience and the right questions are often needed to help them express themselves.

VESTIBULAR LABYRINTH TO VESTIBULAR NUCLEI

The vestibular labyrinth, nerves and nuclei are involved in the detection and analysis of movements of the head, whether they are forwards, backwards, side to side or rotary. Damage to this pathway results in a sense of unreal movement with either the patient or his surroundings apparently moving. It is this illusion of movement that is the important feature permitting the patient's symptoms to be called 'vertigo' and setting it aside from other forms of dizziness. The direction or the type of movement is less important in this respect. It can be, and commonly, is rotary when the patient complains that the room is spinning about him, but it can also be that the surroundings move to and fro, with the ground coming up then receding. Other, less common, sensations of unreal movement can occur, and it is often helpful to provide an example that the patient can compare to his own sensations. One example known to the young, and sometimes not so young, is the sensation that occurs when you step from a playground roundabout that has been spinning. As soon as you reach the ground and stand still, the world about continues to spin around. Of course the world is not spinning, but the endolymph or the otoconia still have momentum and continue to move for a short while stimulating the sensory cells of the labyrinth which are stationary. Most people will have felt this sensation at some time. An alternative example which most medical students seem to have experienced occurs after the rapid consumption of too much alcohol. As they slump into an armchair and close their eyes the room appears to spin round (the 'whirling pit' syndrome). The sensation probably arises as the rate of diffusion of the alcohol into the perilymph and endolymph is different so that the relative density of the two fluids changes very slightly. Movement of the endolymph then occurs with subsequent stimulation of the sensory cells.

The result in both these examples is vertigo which arises because of mis-match of the sensory information arriving at the brainstem. In both cases the vestibular labyrinth is telling the brainstem that the movement is occurring whilst the eyes report that the earth is still and the somatosensors indicate that the body is firmly attached to the ground or the armchair. This confused information results in the individual being aware of apparent but unreal movement. If the stimulus is severe or the person is particularly susceptible, autonomic pathways in the brainstem are stimulated with changes in pulse and blood pressure so that the unfortunate individual becomes pale, clammy, and sweaty and may eventually feel nauseated and vomit (Figure 2.1).

This completed picture is often found in acute disorders of the vestibular labyrinth and nuclei but does not help distinguish the site of the disease as being peripheral (vestibular labyrinth) or central (brainstem vestibular nuclei).

Some additional features may however help in making this important distinction. If the peripheral vestibular disease is not too severe and the false input from the labyrinth not overwhelming it is often possible partly to suppress the unpleasant sensations by increasing the correct input from the eyes and somatosensors, thereby giving the brainstem more information to work on. Patients do this by fixing their gaze hard on a stationary object and by gripping firmly onto a nearby fixture.

Figure 2.1: Diagram of the vestibular system afflicted by disease when additional changes are brought about by the brainstem and symptoms of nausea and 'dizziness' occur.

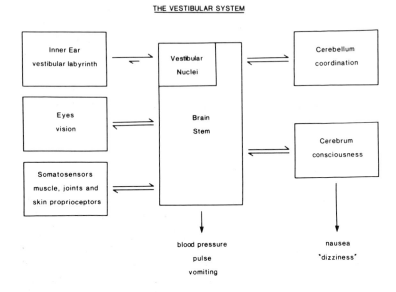

THE VESTIBULAR SYSTEM

This may be just enough to counteract the erroneous laby-rinthine information. When the central brainstem nuclei are disordered, increasing the input often makes no difference and might even make the symptoms worse.

The two examples both involved rotary vertigo with the sufferer feeling that the world was spinning. This is probably the most common sensation described but other directions of move-ment occur. Less frequently patients complain that their head or their whole body is moving, or even that the inside of the head is spinning, or moving to and fro. These sensations get more difficult to describe the further they depart from the classical presentation, but the feature that allows them to be called vertigo is the sense of unreal movement.

Following a definite attack of vertigo whether short or long-lived, many patients continue to feel unsteady, wobbly, or just that things are not quite right with their balance. There appear to be compensatory mechanisms, probably mediated by the cerebellum, at work during this recovery phase, and these, often vague, symptoms are presumably due to incomplete compens-ation. Frequently this unsteadiness is made worse by moving a

14

little too quickly, or changing direction rather suddenly, and sometimes by abrupt changes in what can be seen, such as an action-packed sequence on a wide screen at the cinema, or more simply, a stream of cars passing quickly by. Taken in isolation these symptoms can sometimes appear peculiar but if questioned properly the report of the preceding vertiginous attack allows sense to be made and avoids the label of 'neurotic' being firmly tied to the sufferer. Occasionally, and especially in the elderly, these symptoms persist long after the original vertiginous attack, which may have been forgotten, and makes the diagnostic problem all the more difficult.

POSITIONAL VERTIGO

One form of vertigo can occur with fairly sudden changes of head position, as happens when turning over in bed or when working under the car and turning the head to one side. On the first occasion a rotary vertigo occurs, lasting perhaps a minute or two, and may be severe enough to make the individual feel nauseated but rarely vomit. After some further experiences like this it is realised that only one specific manoeuvre causes the trouble. It may be he has had to turn so that the right ear is down, or it may occur on standing up suddenly with the head turned to the left; the combinations are many but it is always one particular event that causes the problem for the individual. The room really does seem to spin round for a short while and it is usually easy to distinguish these symptoms from those of light-headedness, weakness and even blurred vision that we all know from standing up suddenly after being in the sun for too long, or in a bath of water which is really a bit too hot.

These latter symptoms arise from a short-lived reduction in the blood supply to the brain and are described later in this chapter.

The patient's description of positional vertigo is usually fairly clear-cut, and as we will see later, is most often caused by mischief in the labyrinth. It can, however, arise from disease in the brain and it may not be possible to distinguish the site of the disorder on the symptoms alone. Fortunately the distinction between the two sites can usually be made by a simple clinical testing to be described in Chapter 4.

OSCILLOPSIA

An uncommon but real set of symptoms may arise after the vestibular labyrinths fail completely or are both destroyed, as sometimes occurred when streptomycin was in fashion and as may now happen following treatment with other, newer aminoglycosides. Rarely both vestibular nerves may have been divided either by trauma or surgery or some combination. The vestibular nuclei are therefore deprived of information about the more rapid forms of head movement as occur during walking and running. They have to rely on information from the eyes and from the neck somatosensors about changes in head position to be able to maintain a stable eye position. The information that these two provide is not good enough to compensate for the more rapid changes so that eye fixation is poor. The end result of this is that the patient complains that the surroundings move up and down or bob around when they are walking, running or travelling on the local buses, but not when they are still or travelling in the Rolls Royce. Other directions of apparent movement occur when the head is moved, say from side to side. The effect of this form of oscillopsia can be quite disturbing to patients making them very unsteady and unwilling to move at all quickly.

This symptom is different from the visual effects that commonly occur in the aura prior to an attack of migraine. Blurring, apparent shimmering of objects, moving spots or lines may all occur but are not related to movement and the subsequent headache separates this form of oscillopsia from that of vestibular failure.

Other rarer causes of oscillopsia, albeit with the same symptoms and caused by some centrally induced disorders of eye movement, have been described and are reviewed in an excellent article by Bender (1965).

OCULAR DISORDERS

The rapid development of a paralysis of one or more of the muscles that move the eyes results in a sensation of unreal movement when the sufferer tries to look in different directions or moves his head. The symptoms are worse when the head or eyes are moved in the direction of pull of the paralysed muscle.

They arise because there is a discrepancy between the somato-sensory input from the neck and the visual information received about the location of the target on the retina, or between the information received from each eye. The result is a sense of unreal movement with perhaps the room tilting one way or the other during walking or turning.

The same sensation can be experienced at some fairground sideshows where rooms have been built with a tilting floor yet vertical walls and with window frames not aligned to either. Walking across such a room induces visual-somatosensory mis-match and results in a feeling of an abnormal tilting movement and an associated unsteadiness of gait with a tendency to veer off and fall to one or other side.

Performing tasks involving reaching out to pick up objects is also impaired in people who suddenly develop squints as this requires matching visual and somatosensory inputs. The hand is directed to one or other side of the object depending on which extra ocular muscle is paralysed.

In addition to these symptoms there is frequently double vision, blurred vision or reduced acuity. Fortunately the central pathways usually compensate quickly for the sensory mis-match, at least as far as the vertigo and motor performance are concerned, and eventually even the sensation of diplopia may diminish as the visual input from the affected eye is suppressed so that the blurred vision and poor acuity may also improve.

A transitory vertigo can also be experienced by those people with very poor vision especially following cataract operations who start wearing spectacles with powerful lenses. When they move their eyes to one side or the other, the peripheral parts of the lenses are being used and act as miniature prisms displacing the image from its correct position on the retina (Adler 1941). A sensory mis-match occurs and there is a feeling of movement to one side of the body and an unsteadiness with a slight swaying of the body. The direction of the sense of movement changes from looking one way then the other and in the older person with deteriorating sensation from the legs may result in a fall. Fortunately the use of contact lenses goes a long way to overcoming the problem.

THE SOMATOSENSORS

The various receptors found in the skin, muscles and joints and their sensory nerves can be affected by many disorders with the more common being described in Chapter 16. The occurrence of a peripheral sensory neuropathy frequently results in an unsteadiness as the input to the brainstem becomes inadequate or inaccurate. A frequently associated weakness of the motor nerves and muscles only makes the problems worse as the body finds itself incapable of performing the correct motor response to instructions from the brain. The end results of a severe motor neuropathy is paralysis whilst the sensory neuropathies at an advanced stage tend to cause peripheral pain and loss of sensation. It is the earlier stages of disease that concern us here, when the failing peripheral nerves cannot report positional information quite correctly nor bring about the completely appropriate response. The result is unsteadiness and because of the complexity of the sensory input and motor output descriptions of remarkable ingenuity are often heard.

Commonly the patient feels as if he is walking on cotton wool, or across a soft mattress. Sometimes the pavements are made of rubber or jelly or the knees feel wobbly. When positional information from the eyes is reduced, as in the dark or with failing eyesight, the problems become worse and the patient frequently has to hold onto a rail or even use a walking stick, not only as a support for fear of falling, but also to provide additional sensory information through the somatosensors of the hands and arms. The individual does not faint, for this is a central problem, but may feel the legs go from under him, and sometimes ends up as an embarrassed, ungainly heap on the ground.

The classic description involves the patient bending forwards over a sink with eyes closed about to wash his face. The loss of visual input and a poor somatosensory input means that he is trying to maintain his balance with the vestibular labyrinth alone. This is doomed to failure, as is virtually any attempt to maintain balance with only one of the three vestibular sensations, and the patient ends in the Casualty Department having cracked his head against the sink as he collapses.

To compensate for the difficulties the patient experiences with walking (because of inadequate sensory and motor function) the gait sometimes changes into a waddling, feet more widely spaced, style which gives more stability. This is more often noticed by the doctor than mentioned by the patient, but may be part of the presenting symptoms and is an additional clue to localising the disorder if the description of the unsteadiness is confusing.

THE CEREBELLUM

A large part of the cerebellum is involved with the smooth co-ordination of movement and disease results in the failure to control precisely motor function. The result of this inco-ordination is clumsiness or unsteadiness and in the absence of any muscle weakness is called ataxia.

Ataxia, in the broadest sense, can also result from failure of the sensory input from the eyes, the vestibular labyrinth or the somatosensors, when insufficient information is available to maintain smooth function. It is usually apparent to the patient that his vision has altered and this rarely causes a problem. Acute failure of the vestibular system is nearly always accompanied by vertigo and again usually becomes evident in the patient's story. Loss of peripheral sensory input may give the peculiar sensations described previously. Failure of the cerebellum, however, brings a different set of problems. Disease of one or other side of the cerebellum causes ataxia of the limbs of the same side. The patient feels unsteady and, in addition, not only senses that he is being pulled or pushed over to that side, but actually is. He tends to bump into objects, always on the same side, and veers off to that side when walking. It is only with great difficulty that he manages to walk in a straight line. He may also say that his hand has become clumsy or that it may not work properly so as to have become virtually useless.

Disease of the central portion of the cerebellum is much more severe, especially if acute and can be absolutely disastrous for the patient. In addition to the so-called truncal ataxia when the whole body is unbalanced, but the limbs are spared, there are frequently disorders of speech, swallowing and breathing. The unfortunate individual suffers violent unsteadiness as soon as he tries to sit or stand from being quietly still, and is virtually unable to sit upright unaided. Walking may be quite impossible. This central portion of the cerebellum is closely involved with co-ordinating information from the vestibular labyrinth so he

19

might feel vertiginous and nauseated when trying to move but is usually free from trouble when sitting quietly still. The speech may become broken up into syllables, each being pronounced with great difficulty, or if the effort is too much the words and speech become almost continuous and confused. Added to this is inco-ordination of breathing with the larynx and vocal cords being out of step with the diaphragm and rib cage so that the pitch and volume of speech is altered from moment to moment. There is nearly always a major disruption of eye movement that will be described in the section on examination (Chapter 4).

THE BRAINSTEM

The preceding sections have started to reveal the complexity of the brainstem in the maintenance of normal balance. Many of the interactions between the vestibular labyrinth and nuclei, the eyes, the somatosensors and the cerebellum occur in the brainstem so that disease here can cause vertigo in many forms depending on the location of the damage. The overlap that occurs between the various components within the brainstem means that clear-cut symptoms, as often arise with purely peripheral disease, may not be described with central disorders. However, the hallmark of established brainstem disease is its persistence and the frequent involvement of other functions caused by the tight-packing of important structures in a small space.

The persistence of symptoms almost certainly arises because the protective inhibitory function of the cerebellum that would damp-down the effects of abnormal impulses from say an unhealthy vestibular labyrinth is unable to function correctly because, in this case, the damaged brainstem is not responsive to such inhibition. Additional input from the eyes and somatosensors is also not of much value because the central mechanisms are damaged and cannot make use of what would, in the case of labyrinth failure, be valuable information.

Thus, established disease in the brainstem tends to result in a vertigo that lasts for days and weeks, rather than one or two days as might occur in acute complete labyrinth failure caused by trauma. In this latter case the unsteadiness that occurs whilst compensation is taking place, may persist for a long time, even for ever in the elderly, but the spontaneous illusion of movement has gone after a relatively short while.

Positional vertigo, like that described in the section on the vestibular labyrinth (p. 15) can also occasionally occur with brainstem disease. The symptoms are usually indistinguishable, unless there are additional brainstem features.

When the blood supply to the brainstem is interrupted either transiently or permanently, many additional symptoms can arise as other nuclei and nerve pathways are involved. Table 2.1 shows what symptoms can arise, but vertigo is nearly always top of the list whatever combination occurs.

The exact combination, of course, varies depending on the territories disabled by hypoxia, and so it has been found that these symptoms and the associated signs tend to cluster into a number of loosely defined syndromes that are described more fully in the chapter on brainstem disease (Chapter 14).

THE CEREBRUM

The workings or failings of the cerebrum can effect balance in two ways. First, failure of the blood supply or one of the essential components such as oxygen or glucose can bring about alterations in consciousness sometimes with sensations of dizzi-

Table 2.1: Symptoms associated with interruption of the brainstem blood supply

Dizziness:	Vertigo
	Unsteadiness
	Collapse
	Drop attacks
Vomiting	
Visual defects:	Blurred vision
	Double vision
	Patchy loss of vision
Dysarthria	
Dysphonia	
Dysphagia	
Hiccough	
Paraesthesia:	Uni- or bilateral
	Face/arms/legs
Weakness:	Uni- or bilateral
	Face/arms/legs
Headache	
Confusion	

ness and often with collapse. This group of conditions can be collected under the title of syncope. Second, an altered psyche can prompt feelings of dizziness, sometimes amongst many other symptoms, often as the only complaint.

Syncope

There cannot be many normal people who have not experienced sensations from a transient alteration in blood supply to the brain. Jumping up suddenly after a long time in bed, especially during a bout of influenza may bring on a feeling of light-headedness, of a 'swimmy' sensation in the head, or of feeling slightly inebriated. In addition, the vision may blur or go grey and dim, and the arms and legs feel weak and useless. The legs may even give way and force you back to the bed so that the next time you get up more slowly. This collection of symptoms comes on rapidly, lasts only a short time, recovers completely, and the cause is obvious. Exactly the same symptoms may be brought on by disease and without the need for changes in position. The extent of the alteration in consciousness can of course be more marked with the patient developing a full blown faint, with loss of consciousness, and even, if the lack of blood or oxygen is severe enough, convulsive movements, often to be confused with true epilepsy. These extremes do not really concern us here but the incomplete development of the full attack does. The sensation of light-headedness is frequently called 'vertigo', 'giddiness' or 'dizziness' by patients and does not help the doctor at all. A more exact description of the sensation, perhaps by example, and the association with blurred vision and weakness helps immensely in applying the label 'syncope' so that the cause can be more quickly found. If the legs give way spontaneously without any other apparent sensation then the use of the label 'syncope' is inappropriate and the term drop-attack should be applied. Drop attacks are described in Chapter 17.

Psyche

An individual's personality is made up of a number of distinctive traits or tendencies, which are the ways in which that individual reacts in a set of circumstances. An 'optimist' will respond in one way to an item of news whereas a 'pessimist' will respond in another, possibly opposite way. Personality is therefore a potential possessed by an individual, facets of which may never be expressed if certain conditions do not arise. For example, someone with paranoid traits may fail to show them if their life-style protects them from personal pressure. A personality disorder arises in an individual if he deviates so far away from what is regarded as the normal level of expression of one or more of his own personality traits, that he is liable to exhibit distressing symptoms or behaviour in circumstances when others would not.

The next step up, and sometimes merging with the extremes of the personality disorders, are the neuroses which are emotional responses displayed when an individual is troubled by his environment so that his mood is altered beyond all reasonable limits. For this individual the real world still exists, his personality is intact, he does not have delusions or hallucinations but his mood changes too easily and excessively. This state of affairs is frequently associated with physical symptoms. The neuroses can express themselves in many ways and anxiety, obsessional and paranoid neuroses, like a depressive neurosis or illness, are common. Personality disorders and the neuroses are, in general, responses to changes in either the physical or emotional environment of the patient.

A more severe and less common disorder is a psychosis where there are disturbances of thinking and perception that cannot be explained simply as a response to some environmental change. This form of disorder is severe enough to distort the individual's appreciation and judgement of the real world and relationships within it. Hallucinations and delusions are common.

A rather special and perhaps quite different condition is hysteria which can be loosely described as a disturbance of behaviour whereby symptoms and signs of physical ill-health are imitated more or less unconsciously for some sort of personal gain. Hysteria is, not surprisingly, a frequently misused term (Slater 1965) and the condition is not merely an extension in severity of the hysterical personality. Although some patients with hysteria have an underlying hysterical personality, the term conversion hysteria or conversion reaction better illustrates that hysteria is one particular reaction to a distressing emotional experience. However, in many series patients who had received the label 'hysteria', had an underlying organic disease often diagnosed much later or by the pathologist at post-mortem. Physical disease can thus present as hysteria before specific symptoms and signs of that disease are apparent. Thus, hysteria can be a reaction to an overwhelming pressure such as a depressive illness or as occurs on the battlefield, or be a response to a hidden organic disease, thereby illustrating the complex intertwining of mind and body.

Vertigo is a frequent expression of conversion hysteria (Trimble 1981) but pure hysterical vertigo is seldom encountered and careful examination almost always reveals some underlying vestibular abnormality (Dix 1973).

Patients with more common disorders of the psyche often have physical symptoms, and frequently attend a medical or surgical clinic. Some of these patients will be dizzy, and whilst it is not usually necessary for us to make a precise diagnosis of the psychiatric condition, it is important to realise that behind the frequently peculiar descriptions of their unsteadiness lies mental ill-health that, if correctly managed, could remove the presenting features. The problem is to be aware that this can occur and yet not label any undiagnosed case of dizziness as psychiatric.

An anxiety neurosis frequently presents with bouts of vertigo, usually short-lived, but often associated with panic attacks. Generalised unsteadiness frequently surrounds the acute attacks which may be set off by any unsettling occurrence. Other symptoms arising from the anxiety accompany the dizziness. A dry mouth, tingling sensations, especially of the lips and fingers, palpitations, choking sensations and a 'queasy' stomach may all be present if asked about, but the picture may be clouded if the patient hyperventilates and brings on a syncopal attack.

The overt depressive illnesses appear to be less commonly associated with dizziness but masked depression often shows itself by physical symptoms, one of which is frequently dizziness, unsteadiness or a fear of collapse. These symptoms may be very difficult for the patient to describe and cannot really be likened to any sensation experienced in the past. A persisting and overwhelming pre-occupation with dizziness may suggest an attempt at malingering but is more often an expression of an underlying depression.

3

The History

Taking a proper history is really the key to diagnosing dizziness but to do this requires that you should know the possible causes and their associated symptoms so that a realistic set of questions can be posed. There is really little point in taking a detailed dietary history for a possible vitamin deficiency anaemia if the patient has a rotary vertigo that lasts for hours rather than a transient light-headedness on standing up. This chapter therefore should come at the end of the book but then the format of the time-honoured clinical method of history, examination and investigation is lost. Perhaps the best thing to do is to re-read this chapter when you are more familiar with the range of conditions that cause dizziness.

The first, and often the hardest, step is to find out what is the sensation that is causing concern. I have tried to describe the variety of forms that dizziness can take in Chapter 2, and have outlined the major conditions that affect the various parts of the system later in the book. Now I will attempt to provide a framework for reaching a likely diagnosis that can be confirmed or refuted by the examination and investigations. Broadly speaking the large variety of different symptoms can be allocated to one of four major groups, which I am going to call: (1) vertigo; (2) unsteadiness; (3) light-headedness and (4) giddiness. There is often overlap and frequently an individual's symptoms may fall into several groups. Nevertheless the reason for attempting this allocation is to pick out first of all that group of patients with vertigo, as they often have a clear-cut history that conforms to a recognisable pattern. They may also have additional symptoms of unsteadiness and light-headedness but the presence of the illusion of movement points to disorder in one relatively limited portion of the vestibular system.

Unsteadiness is a less clearly defined, but large group containing all those conditions affecting the somatosensors, the muscles and joints, occasionally the eyes and sometimes intracranial structures. There is, however, no illusion of movement, any movement that does occur being real. Unsteadiness can occur when the vertigo that follows, say, a head injury has settled and the central mechanisms are compensating, although here the past history gives the clue.

Light-headedness is a little easier as it usually comes quite well-defined by the patient who, more likely than not, has experienced the same sensation as a 'normal' event at some time in their life.

The giddy ones are the more difficult. Patients have symptoms they cannot easily define or describe but which seem real to them although perhaps bizarre to you. You might be tempted to label these as psychiatric, and indeed some of them will be, but you should only do this when you have excluded underlying organic disease.

VERTIGO

Most of the patients complaining of vertigo will have something wrong with their ears. A few will have trouble with the brainstem and its connections or with their eyes.

The quality of the vertigo should be explored first. Do the surroundings appear to move or is it the patient who is in apparent motion? The events surrounding the onset of the first attack may make the diagnosis obvious. For example, was there a head injury or trauma to the neck, say, in a car crash? Did the vertigo arise after diving into water or poking a cotton bud into the ear? Has an operation been performed on the ear recently or some time ago since vertigo can often arise as an acute or delayed complication of middle ear surgery.

How long do the attacks last? Although you can never say never in medicine, vertigo that persists remorselessly for 36 or more hours is never caused by disease in the labyrinth. Something central is wrong. Do the bouts of vertigo occur randomly or do they come on in groups with long intervals free of trouble between the clusters of attacks? Are they associated with periods in female patients?

Most vertigo is made worse by movement so that patients prefer to lie still but, in general, vertigo brought on by changes in position is likely to be caused by disease in the labyrinth, or disorder in the neck or vertebro-basilar arteries. Is the sensation of movement improved with eyes open or closed? Visual fixation often helps lessen a labyrinthine vertigo if it is not too severe. Does the patient lose consciousness? Although an acute labyrinthine vertigo may throw the patient to the floor by its severity, unconsciousness does not occur and its presence strongly suggests that something is amiss with the brain or its blood supply, and you should ask about features suggestive of epilepsy.

Is there a warning of the attack, with a feeling of fullness in the ear, perhaps a change in the hearing or the development of, or a change in an already existing tinnitus. These features point to a labyrinthine cause for the vertigo whilst a preceding viral-type illness, perhaps an upper respiratory tract infection, a common cold, a rash or swelling around the ear, contact with chicken-pox or shingles suggest involvement of the vestibular nerve, its ganglion or nucleus.

Apart from the vertigo, the cardinal symptoms of ear disease are: deafness, pain, discharge, tinnitus and facial weakness, and all those must be asked for and followed up if present.

Other symptoms relating to central disease should now be sought if there is no suggestion of labyrinthine disorder. Although it is generally taught that you should not ask leading questions, I think that here you must, since many symptoms may have been forgotten or thought to be too trivial to be mentioned. Perhaps this is especially so for disseminated sclerosis where transient, often painful, loss of vision in one eye, or double vision, a clumsy hand or dragging foot might not be mentioned unless specifically asked for. Separate disturbances of vision such as rapid deterioration of acuity, field defects, 'greying' or total temporary loss of vision point towards disorders of the eye, the attached muscles or central connections, all of which cause or can be associated with the vertigo.

The list of symptoms associated with intracranial disorders is almost endless but the more relevant ones associated with vertigo are pain or numbness in the face (V), difficulty in swallowing, hoarseness or a weak voice (IX and X), difficulty with speaking (IX, X and XII) and headache. This last symptom may well be part of a migrainous disturbance that the patient

27

has suffered for some while and does not associate with the vertigo that can arise when the basilar artery and its branches are involved.

If you now suspect that there is something going on in the brainstem that is not multiple sclerosis or migraine, an embolus from a cancer especially of the lung, stomach or breast, or from a diseased heart valve will be high on your list of suspicions and so the relevant questions should be posed.

At some time you must also find out what medications the patient is taking or has received in the past as there are a number of drugs (described in Chapter 11) with specific vestibulototoxic side-effects.

UNSTEADINESS

Once vertigo has been excluded as a symptom and you have decided that unsteadiness is the problem, it now becomes important to decide whether the sensation is associated with real movement and a tendency to fall or veer away to one side, or whether there is just a feeling of 'wobbliness', of walking on cotton wool or some similarly expressed difficulty often associated with a non-specific instability. You must then exclude pure muscle weakess — as might arise following recovery from a stroke — or joint pain and stiffness as causing the trouble. Often patients find difficulty in distinguishing between weakness and clumsiness but a lessened ability to push themselves up out of an armchair is a reasonably good indicator of weakness. Of course, the picture is frequently not clear-cut, and you have to decide whether a small degree of weakness or a stiff hip is enough to account for all their symptoms.

In the first group — those with a tendency to topple to one side — the majority of causes arise from intracranial disease affecting the brainstem or cerebellum. The symptoms tend to come on in their completed form, either because a sudden event like a bleed or an embolus occurred or because a slowly progressive disease such as a tumour compressing the brainstem finally overcomes the compensatory mechanisms. It is unusual for there to be no associated symptoms although ataxia like this may sometimes be the first presenting feature in disseminated sclerosis (multiple sclerosis). Nevertheless, you must ask about previous symptoms suggestive of disseminated sclerosis, especially in the younger age groups, and about symptoms suggestive of other acute troubles in the brainstem and its connections caused by a bleed or embolus. If the answers are suggestive of something embolic then once more cancers of the lung, stomach and breast or defective heart valves are a frequent source and the relevant questions should be posed.

Tumours growing in the cerebello-pontine angle are not all that rare and sometimes present with ataxia. They are usually benign and are frequently found on the vestibular nerve (although they are called acoustic neuromas). There is nearly always a profound hearing loss associated with these and the other tumours of this region, and this loss although usually progressive can be sudden in onset.

The second group, comprising those with a feeling of unsteadiness and perhaps a diffuse instability compensated for by an altered gait, is much larger with many possible causes. The majority, however, will have some defect of the peripheral sensory nerves so that the somatosensory input is inadequate for normal balance.

Ask whether they are being treated for diabetes or if not, whether they get very thirsty and pass a lot of urine. Perhaps they have noticed a recent need to get up at night to empty their bladder. A combination of weight loss and increased appetite is suspicious as is the development of recurrent bouts of itching and irritation, especially of the vulva. Pruritus is also common in chronic uraemia, another cause of peripheral neuropathy. Here there is frequently increased pigmentation in an otherwise dry flaky skin, so that with the anaemia which is nearly universal in these patients they tend to develop a sallow unhealthy complexion. Nocturia is also common and if the uraemia is associated with hypertension, the fluid load can produce nocturnal dyspnoea, both of which should be asked about specifically.

Alcoholism, not often admitted to, frequently plays a part and if you are making a home visit, and the opportunity arises, look around to see if the dustbin is full of empty sherry bottles or the like. The alcoholic is resentful of advice, may blame his drinking on others or 'the circumstances', and tends to be forgetful, unreliable and quarrelsome. He may have alcoholic amnesia, remembering nothing after two or three drinks, then waking up hours or days later, finding himself in a strange place, not knowing how he got there. None of this may be admitted but ask about complaints of aching, coldness, hotness, numbness or prickling in the calves, feet or fingers. Excessive sweating of hands and feet may develop and the skin of the calves become dry, red and shiny. Alcohol is by far the most common cause of a B-vitamin deficiency neuropathy and it is very uncommon for even severe malnutrition to cause this problem.

However, a number of drugs do and so you must make full enquiry into present and past medication, and also about exposure to mercury and lead compounds — especially the organic mercurials. Other organic chemicals like cleaning fluids and various solvents occasionally cause problems and so you should ask if the patient comes into contact with such things in the course of their work or hobbies.

Syphilis, like alcoholism, is frequently not admitted, yet can cause a sensory neuropathy often selectively affecting the somatosensory input. You should question directly but perhaps you can ask whether they have received courses of injections for social disease, venereal disease, sexually transmitted disease or whatever phrase you feel happy with that is not too obscure. Although late syphilis almost certainly does not occur with appropriate and adequate treatment of the early disease, a number of patients still slip through the net and present with late symptoms.

Sometimes problems with the spinal cord from compression, stretching, infiltration or trauma will cause a combination of sensory loss and weakness in the legs. Impotence, abnormalities of bladder and bowel function may occur in combination with the unsteadiness and should certainly be asked for specifically as once again patients may be too shy or embarrassed to tell all when asked the question 'do you have any other problems?'

You may well have drawn no helpful answers from such a series of questions and then the possibility arises that the patient has a hidden carcinoma, usually of the lung or ovary, but occasionally of the gut, that is causing a peripheral neuropathy that is not metastatic in origin. Rarely the neuropathy is purely sensory when the unsteadiness may be associated with shooting pains, but more commonly there is additional slight weakness. Carcinoma must therefore be suspected especially in middle and later life and enquiry made about smoking, cough, haemoptysis and weight loss. A change in bowel habit with constipation or diarrhoea, the presence of blood or mucus give cause for further questioning and direction to the subsequent examination and investigations. Symptoms of ovarian carcinoma are uncommon until a complication occurs. The symptoms that do occur are enlargement of the abdomen, a sense of fullness and a bearing down discomfort in the pelvis, pressure effects on the bladder or rectum with frequency and constipation respectively, and varicosites or oedema of the leg because of obstruction of the venous return or lymphatic drainage. Pain is rare.

The bronchogenic and ovarian carcinomas can also give rise to a cerebellar degeneration where the ataxia is much more profound and the gait changes markedly although there is usually no trouble with arm movements. Unsteadiness and gross ataxia can also be caused by a prolonged and excessive intake of alcohol and less commonly by exposure to the heavy metals, all of which cause varying degrees of degeneration and cell loss in the cerebellum.

More widespread cell loss occurs in the less common spino-cerebellar degenerations which are usually hereditary but may arise sporadically. As well as the unsteadiness and ataxia many other symptoms arise depending on the extent and site of the degenerative processes. The various manifestations of the disease arise at different ages with a range of forms of present-ation that have been allocated a baffling variety of names — over fifty syndromes are to be found in the literature. Neverthe-less, there is frequently a family history of a similar disturbance and the condition often presents with unsteadiness then stumb-ling and awkwardness progressing to gross ataxia.

LIGHT-HEADEDNESS

The circumstances surrounding the onset of light-headedness are most important as a guide to sorting out the cause of the trouble. You must therefore find out by questioning whether the faintness comes on during a change of position from lying or sitting to standing up, or whether it occurs spontaneously even when the patient is lying down. Occasionally the circumstances guide you directly to an answer if the patient reports that the symptoms occur following a prolonged bout of coughing or during the night when he gets up to urinate. Less easy circum-stances surround the very common hyperventilation syndrome which is nearly always a manifestation of acute anxiety,

31

although the sufferer may not be aware of the overbreathing. These patients, in addition to the light-headedness, report tightness in the chest and throat, and feelings of suffocation or of impending doom. Tingling, numbness or coldness of lips, fingers and toes almost confirms the diagnosis.

The first group mentioned — those with a postural light-headedness — have a transient inadequacy of the blood supply to the cerebrum. Some of these are caused by an idiopathic disorder of the autonomic nervous system where there is failure of the reflex peripheral vasoconstriction on standing up. This is often associated with impotence, bladder problems and loss of sweating in the legs. However, a number of other conditions that need specific management also cause postural light-headedness. You must therefore find out if the patient is being treated for high blood pressure or has recently changed his tablets for a different type as an overdose or inappropriate medication can be the culprit.

Ask about symptoms of anaemia. Tiredness, weakness, lack of energy and shortness of breath all lead you in the right direction and should prompt you to delve deeper into the background of the condition.

Is the patient being treated for diabetes? Occasionally an autonomic neuropathy can occur causing a failure of the postural vascular compensation. If they are not being treated, are there any other symptoms suggestive of the condition? Syphilis in its later stages can also produce the same autonomic neuropathy and depending on your rapport with the patient should be enquired about as described before.

Inappropriate treatment of diabetes can result in attacks of hypoglycaemia, with light-headedness as the predominant feature, and this introduces us to the second group where the symptoms can occur without postural change. Hypoglycaemia may arise following major gastric surgery as a 'dumping' syndrome where faintness occurs some hours after a heavy meal. The same symptoms occur after fasting or exercise in patients with the rare insulin-producing tumours of the pancreas, and occasionally in Addison's disease where the malaise and weakness, typical of anaemia are accompanied by a dusky pigmentation like a sun-tan that just will not wash off.

The majority of this group, however, will probably have some cardiovascular problem. You should ask about palpitations, whether they occur and if they do, whether they are fast or slow, regular or irregular. Has the patient had heart disease diagnosed in the past, perhaps a heart attack or valve disorder, especially aortic stenosis? Is the light-headedness associated with chest pain or physical exertion; does the patient have a pacemaker in place? The answers to these questions can lead you towards a tentative diagnosis that will be settled later on by your examination and subsequent investigations.

GIDDINESS

This final group is perhaps the most difficult as the quality of the dizziness does not fall into any easily recognisable pattern. The patient may be unable to express the sensation but is usually certain that it is not vertigo, unsteadiness or pure light-headedness when examples are given. The sensations described include continuous non-specific disorientation, bouts of fear of falling, attacks of 'confusion in the head' — the list is almost endless, frequently bizarre and can immediately suggest that the patient is mad. There is no best word to describe these sensations but giddiness is useful when it is defined as not vertigo, not unsteadiness and not light-headedness. Matthews' comments now seem very appropriate 'There can be few physicians so dedicated to their art that they do not experience a slight decline in spirits on learning that their patient's complaint is giddiness' (Matthews 1970). In spite of this you must not despair for you will be able to help some people or perhaps direct them to those who can.

Ask about when the symptoms come on and what else accompanies them. A longstanding continuous giddiness that persists day in, day out without any other features is most difficult to assess and is frequently a manifestation of a longstanding anxiety state that can be intractable. Bouts of giddiness are more accessible to enquiry. Some are associated with ear symptoms — deafness, tinnitus, pain or discharge — and may settle when the ear is treated, although the precise cause of the upset is never found. Many of the rest will have giddiness as part of a generalised anxiety which is often a component of a number of psychiatric and organic conditions. Commonly associated symptoms are apprehension, fear of impending disaster or disease, irritability, sweating, tremor, choking sensations, or lump in the throat and palpitations. The patient may also hyperventilate and become light-headed and this part of the history helps lead you to the underlying anxiety.

Some of the symptoms of acute anxiety, including giddiness, can occur from underlying organic disease. Thyrotoxicosis, paroxysmal tachycardia, hypoglycaemic attacks, toxic confusional states and the rare phaeochromocytomas are all good candidates so the relevant questions should be asked.

Epilepsy presents as transient episodes of disturbed physical function, consciousness or thinking or some combination of these three. Any part of the brain can be involved so that a wide variety of symptoms can develop. The form that is most familiar is a loss of consciousness followed by a fit. This may be heralded by an aura but in many the aura and loss of consciousness are all that occurs. In others the aura may exist alone, but in all cases the contents of the aura suggests the site of instability in the brain and perhaps the location of underlying disease. With focal epilepsy a variety of sensations can be produced and giddiness is frequent amongst them. If it is followed by a collapse through loss of consciousness then often the giddiness is blamed for the collapse. The unconsciousness is important since it indicates that something has happened to the brain and this feature must be carefully assessed if not from the patient then from a relative or friend.

More difficult to evaluate are those that remain conscious and have only an aura. Other hallucinations may accompany the giddiness. Strange feelings in the abdomen or chest, spontaneous and unprovoked tastes and smells, occasionally visual hallucinations can all occur, and although sometimes difficult to separate from the sensations that arise in an anxiety state, especially in an articulate patient, help suggest a focal epilepsy.

By the end of the history taking you should have a good idea where the problem lies and your subsequent examination can be directed towards this part of the vestibular system. Sometimes, even though you do not suspect any underlying disease, it will be necessary to perform a wide-ranging examination for two reasons: first to satisfy yourself, and second, and more importantly, as reassurance for the anxious patient that there is nothing seriously wrong.

4

The Examination and Investigations

The vestibular system is rather like a can of worms. Touch one worm and they all move — stimulate or destroy one section of the vestibular system and many reactions and compensations occur. These features allow us to observe the effects of disease and test the function that remains. As mentioned in the first chapter, the vestibular system has two main roles; to maintain eye-position and to keep us standing upright and co-ordinated. These two functions provide the pathway to testing vestibular function by watching spontaneous or induced eye movements, and by observing stance, gait and co-ordination. These procedures will be described first and then the rest of the neurological examination explained.

NYSTAGMUS

Little else seems to bring a louder groan from medical students than the mere mention of nystagmus. This probably occurs because it can be made into a difficult subject by involving complex and poorly understood central pathways in an attempt to explain what is happening to the eyes. Many types of nystagmus are exceedingly rare and here we will only deal with the more commonly seen forms which provide a very useful diagnostic aid to examining the vestibular system. But a warning first: nystagmus is like virtually all other neurological signs in that it can tell us if something is wrong, it may sometimes tell us where the trouble is, but it can never tell us what the disease is.

Nystagmus is a rhythmic oscillating movement of the eyes, that is for all intents and purposes involuntary, and involves both eyes. It derives from the Greek term meaning sleepy and is supposed to suggest the pattern of eye movement by allusion to the movement of the head that occurs as you are nodding off to sleep. The head slowly sinks towards your chest as your eyes close and then at the last moment jerks rapidly back as your eyes open and you realise you were on the brink of falling asleep.

This slow drift and a rapid flick back is the form of eye movement that may sometimes be seen with disorders of the vestibular labyrinth, nerve and nuclei. It is the slow drift that is the abnormal part and the fast flick that is the normal movement trying to restore eye position. Unfortunately, the direction of the nystagmus has conventionally been named after the direction of the fast phase which is easy to see, whilst it is the slow phase that gives more information. Nystagmus of this form can be from side to side (horizontal), up and down (vertical) or rotary with sometimes a small overlap so that, say, a strong rotary nystagmus has a small horizontal component in it (Figure 4.1).

Figure 4.1: Diagram illustrating the three types of nystagmus. When looking at the patient the rapid phase in both the horizontal and rotary nystagmus is to the patient's left so the nystagmus is called left beating horizontal or rotary nystagmus. With the vertical nystagmus the rapid phase is downwards so the nystagmus is 'down-beating'.

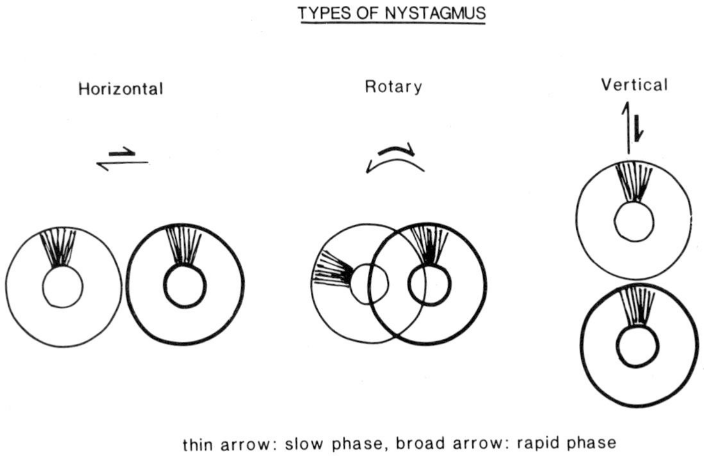

TYPES OF NYSTAGMUS

Horizontal   Rotary   Vertical

thin arrow: slow phase, broad arrow: rapid phase

Nystagmus can also occur when the oscillations are of more or less equal speed in both directions. This is pendular or 'jelly' nystagmus and usually occurs with ocular disorders which will be described later. For the moment we will concentrate on the nystagmus that is typical of disorders of the labyrinth and vestibular nuclei and call it 'vestibular nystagmus' as this is a commonly used term although as we will see not strictly accurate. Another name found in the literature is jerk nystagmus. Vestibular nystagmus can be physiological, spontaneous or induced.

Physiological nystagmus

This can be seen by looking at the eyes of someone who is staring out of a railway carriage window as it is passing a line of telegraph poles. The eyes drift then flick back in rapid succession in the horizontal plane. Vision is fixed first on one of the poles and lateral movement of the eyes keeps this image steady until the eyes reach the limit of their movement when a quick flick returns them more or less to the centre and vision fixes on the next pole. During the quick flick — the saccade — vision is suppressed so that a blurred image is not formed. This is important as the effect of failure of visual suppression can be distressing as you can see for yourself by rapidly, but gently, tapping the very lateral part of the eye, thereby mimicking saccadic movements. The same sort of reflex eye movements occurring in a vertical plane can also be seen in passengers in an old-fashioned lift with a see-through trellis-like door.

This form of physiological nystagmus is properly called optokinetic nystagmus. It is not a product of the vestibular labyrinth and nuclei, but a description has crept in here so that at least we are familiar with the sort of eye movement that can occur in disease.

Spontaneous vestibular nystagmus

Spontaneous nystagmus of a vestibular type always indicates disease when properly observed. To do this the patient is seated in a well-lit position and asked to look straight ahead. He should look at one of your fingers held in front of his face, but

37

not so close that he has to squint to see it. Then ask him to follow your finger as you move it to one side. You must not move the finger so far that the edge of the iris passes the angle of the eye, as at extremes of gaze there may be slight physiological nystagmus because the ocular muscles are at the very limit of their extension or contraction. Do not move the finger very quickly as even in normals this can induce a jerk as the eye reaches its resting position. Observe the eyes closely, then slowly move the finger to the other side, observing the eyes as they move. Have you seen any horizontal or rotary vestibular nystagmus? If you have then there are a few features to note: is the fast phase the same in each direction of eye movement, i.e. does it flick in the same direction on looking both to the left or right or does the direction change? Are both the eyes doing exactly the same thing or are their movements dissociated. If you have seen the patient before, has the nystagmus noticed at previous visit persisted? Is the nystagmus only present when looking in the direction of fast phase (first degree), when looking straight ahead (second phase) or when looking in the direction of the slow phase (third degree)? The same manoeuvres and observations should now be made in the vertical plane moving the eyes up and down. This is more difficult to observe because the eyelids tend to get in the way but the presence of spontaneous vertical nystagmus is important for it indicates central disease. The differentiation between peripheral, that is labyrinthine disorders, and central disease is laid out in Tables 4.1, 4.2 and 4.3.

Table 4.1: Classification of spontaneous horizontal nystagmus

	1st degree	2nd degree	3rd degree
Nystagmus present when:	eyes deviated in direction of fast phase	eyes central	eyes deviated away from direction of fast phase

Localisation of type of disorder

	Peripheral		Central
Combinations	1st degree or 1st and 2nd degree or 1st, 2nd and 3rd degree		some other combination
Magnitude of nystagmus	1st > 2nd > 3rd		some other combination

Table 4.2: Nystagmus: differentiation between peripheral and central disease

	Peripheral	Central
Duration	Temporary Never more than 2 or 3 weeks	Persisting
Direction	Fast phase always the same direction in any eye position	Fast phase may change direction in different eye position
Character	Both eyes move in the same fashion	May be dissociated eye movements
Effects of removing fixation:		
(1) Darkness	Nystagmus enhanced	(i) Vestibular nuclei: enhanced amplitude; frequency declines
		(ii) Above vestibular nuclei: nystagmus abolished
(2) Eyes closed	Nystagmus enhanced	(i) Vestibular nuclei: nystagmus abolished
		(ii) Above vestibular nuclei: nystagmus abolished

Table 4.3: Localisation of various types of nystagmus

	Type of nystagmus		
	Horizontal	Rotary	Vertical
Disorder:			
Peripheral	Often	Often	NEVER
Central	Often	Often	ALWAYS

The last feature in Table 4.2 is the effect of removing fixation on the quality of the nystagmus.

During the basic test we have been asking the patient to focus on our finger. This is providing a visual input which will help suppress the nystagmus caused by a labyrinthine disorder by providing additional information for the brainstem nuclei. If we can remove the visual fixation an enhanced spontaneous nystagmus strongly suggests a labyrinthine disorder. When the central nuclei are diseased removing the visual input may make no difference to the nystagmus, may slow it down (vestibular nuclei) or even reduce or reverse it (other central lesions) as the disordered nuclei have less information to handle. There are several ways of removing fixation. The most obvious is to do the tests in the dark and devise a way of observing eye movement. Several methods have been developed. An infra-red viewer is one easy and expensive answer. Another is to make use of the normal electrical potential that exists across the eyeball from front to back. If electrodes are placed at the corner of each eyeball with a central reference electrode the direction and speed of eye movement can be detected by the changes in potential that occur between the electrodes. This is called electronystagmography (ENG) or more correctly electroculography (EOG) as the technique really measures changes in eye position, one form of which may be nystagmus. Various machines, dedicated to recording such eye movements are available but it is quite possible to use an electrocardiograph (ECG) monitor for the same purpose by having three of the leads to act as the electrodes. A bit of practice is required and the sensitivity of the machine needs to be turned up but it is not too difficult.

An alternative way of removing fixation is to place some very powerful lenses in front of the eyes so that the patient cannot fixate as he is unable to focus, whilst his eyes can still be seen by the examiner. Such a set of spectacles with a dim light behind the lenses so that the eyes can be seen more easily are available under the name of Frenzel's glasses. These glasses are often to be found in a wooden box languishing forgotten in the back of store cupboards. They are very useful as the lenses can be lifted up and down, so making any changes in the intensity of the nystagmus easy to see (Figure 4.2).

If none of this is available then nearly everyone has an ophthalmoscope that can also be used to assess the effects of removal of fixation. Get the patient to look at a distant object in the light, and use the ophthalmoscope to observe the edge of the moving optic disk. Ask someone to switch off the lights so that the room is dark whilst you continue to look at the retina — with luck the movements will change as fixation is abolished. This technique requires some practice, a room that can be made dark and someone else to turn off the lights but needs no 'high technology' aids.

Observing spontaneous nystagmus is difficult, especially at first, but it is worth the effort since a lot of useful information can be gathered with the minimum of fuss. It is also worth looking for spontaneous nystagmus in the absence of fixation since

Figure 4.2: A pair of Frenzel's glasses with the battery carrier for the illumination which lies behind the powerful convex lenses. The patient cannot focus on anything but the observer has a magnified view of the eye.

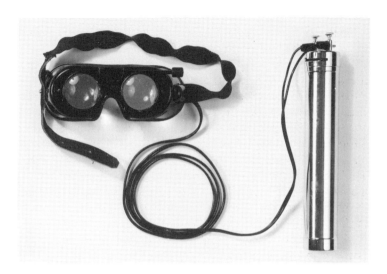

compensation often occurs with peripheral lesions in the light and removing fixation might unmask the nystagmus. The ophthalmoscope is useful for this.

Induced nystagmus

As well as arising spontaneously, vestibular nystagmus can be induced by several test procedures. Many of these require complex equipment, the results are often equivocal, and for the purposes of our examination need bother us no more. Two simple procedures are available which, in combination with the history and the rest of the examination, usually provide enough information to tell us whether something is wrong that needs further attention. These two procedures are positional testing and caloric testing.

POSITIONAL NYSTAGMUS

In the chapter on symptoms, positional vertigo with certain specific head positions inducing a transitory, usually rotary vertigo was mentioned. Positional testing to elicit these symptoms is a must, and, since the test is so easy to perform, should probably be performed on anyone with symptoms of unsteadiness, as it can uncover important pathology.

For this you need a couch and a well-lit room. Sit the patient on the couch so that if they were to lie down their head would hang over the end. Do not lie them down to judge the distance as this may abolish the nystagmus when you get on to doing the test properly. Then, stand at one side of the couch and gently turn the patient's head towards you, asking them to stare at the bridge of your nose. Tell them you are going to lie them down so that their head is hanging down just a little but that you are going to be holding on to their head so that there is no need to be afraid. Then take hold of their head in both hands and as quickly as possible lie them down and let the head hang over the end (Figure 4.3).

Ask them to keep their eyes open and to keep on looking straight at the bridge of your nose. As you are doing all this keep a close watch on their eyes and look for nystagmus. If it arises, is there a delay in its onset, what sort of nystagmus is it, does it adapt, that is fade away after a few seconds, or does it persist while the position is being held? Do they feel vertiginous and if they do, is it the same sort of sensation as their complaint? You may not see any nystagmus, so count to 20 and then sit the patient up, still watching their eyes, and still with the patient's head turned towards you. Does any nystagmus occur on this manoeuvre? If no nystagmus has occurred on this side, then give them a short rest, go to the other side of the couch, and repeat the test with the head turned towards you again.

If nystagmus has occurred when the head was down then repeat the manoeuvre and see if the nystagmus is less severe or the same. It may have disappeared on this second test or be very much diminished. If it is less marked and a further repeat of procedure shows the nystagmus to be negligible or absent then it is said to 'fatigue'. Having decided this then give the patient a rest and go round to test the other side. Abolishing fixation with Frenzel's glasses or ENG during this test seems only to add confusion to the results. By the end of the test you should have

Figure 4.3: (a) The beginning of the positional test. The patient should be staring at the bridge of the tester's nose so that her eyes do not move around. Turn the head gently and wait to ensure that no nystagmus develops from alteration in neck position.
(b) The patient is then rapidly laid down so that her head hangs down over the edge of the couch, whilst still staring at the examiner's face.

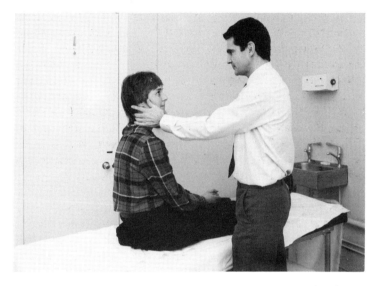

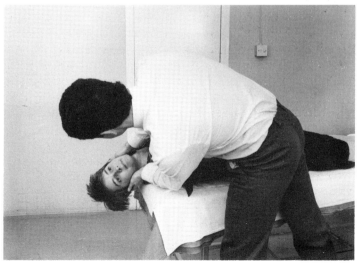

examined both sides and be able to make judgements about the nystagmus under these headings: latency of onset, associated vertigo, adaptation, presence of fatigue, quality of nystagmus, one or both sides.

Two major patterns emerge from this collection of features: benign positional nystagmus and central positional nystagmus (Table 4.4).

The criteria for benign positional nystagmus are quite strict and if fulfilled indicate a condition called benign paroxysmal positional vertigo (BPPV), where the defect is thought to be in the labyrinth and which will be described later in the book. The number of patients with all the signs of benign positional nystagmus who in fact have central disease is diminishingly small. But patients with any deviation from this pattern of benign positional nystagmus quite possibly have central disease whilst those with the features of central positional nystagmus almost certainly do. The complete absence of vertigo in the presence of quite alarming nystagmus is a feature which is often seen in this group, and is a strong pointer to mischief in the brain. Like most things medical, there always appears to be an exception to the rule and in this case the culprit is the demon drink. When the blood alcohol is rising positional alcohol nystagmus phase 1 (PAN1) is found. In the test nystagmus occurs on both sides and is horizontal, with the fast phase towards the lowermost ear, that is, the direction of the nystagmus changes. As the levels of alcohol in endolymph and perilymph equilibrate PAN1 diminishes. Then, as the level of the blood alcohol decreases some 5–6 hours after the drinking session is over, and there are again changes in the distribution of

Table 4.4: Features of positional nystagmus

	Benign	Central
Latent interval	Yes	No
Associated vertigo	Yes	Possible but uncommon
Type of nystagmus	Rotary (often with horizontal component)	Any type
Direction of nystagmus	Towards lowermost ear	Any way
Adaptation	Yes	No
Fatigues	Yes	No
Sides	One only	Often both

alcohol in perilymph and endolymph, PAN2 makes its appearance. Here the nystagmus is away from the lower ear on each side.

There is a lot of individual variation as to the blood alcohol levels needed to induce PAN1, but the more they drink the worse it is. PAN2 is often present when blood alcohol is undetectable and persists for several hours after the last trace of alcohol has gone from the blood, but can be suppressed by drinking more (Aschan, Bergstedt and Stahle 1956; Aschan 1958). This is probably part of the explanation of the efficiency of a pick-me-up (hair of the dog) during a hangover. PAN can cause confusion and so it is a wise procedure to ask directly about when the last drink was taken, perhaps check the blood alcohol level and, if possible repeat the test when they are 'dry', before deciding that the patient has central disease.

CALORIC NYSTAGMUS

The resting output of the vestibular labyrinth of one ear can be stimulated or suppressed by irrigating the ear canal with either warm or cool water. This has the effect of warming or cooling the fluids in the lateral semicircular canal which is the canal closest to the surface of the head. The density of the endolymph therefore alters a little and currents are set up, stimulating the sensory cells of this canal, when no head movement is in fact taking place. The brainstem nuclei therefore receives conflicting information from the two ears and the result is nystagmus and vertigo. With warm water stimulating one labyrinth, the eyes are slowly driven away from that side, and then there is a compensatory flick back, i.e. the nystagmus is to the same side as the irrigation. With cool water the pattern is reversed and nystagmus away from the irrigated ear occurs as the eyes are slowly pushed towards the under-active cool ear by the normal side. The way to remember the directions quickly is to adopt a mnemonic and ACTH (away cold, towards hot) or COWS (cold opposite — warm same) are favourites if only you can remember what the letters stand for.

In a normal subject the nystagmus that results from the irrigation of one ear is more or less equal in intensity and duration to that arising from the other. These reactions form the basis of the caloric tests which are still the best way of testing the function of each labyrinth separately.

As you might imagine the test procedure can be made as simple or as complex as you wish, especially if the effects of removing visual fixation are assessed by doing the tests in the dark with electronystagmography recording eye movement. However, relatively simple procedures have stood the test of time and often provide more than enough information.

Cool caloric testing

The simplest procedure is a cool caloric test. To perform this, first check that there is no large collecion of wax in the ear canal and that there is no perforation in the ear drum, then lie the patient on a couch with the head and body raised up about 30° (Figure 4.4). This brings the horizontal semicircular canal into the vertical position and makes the test more sensitive.

Put an apron or towels round the patient's neck, and have a bowl ready to catch the water that comes out of the ear. The idea of the test is not to induce violent nystagmus with vertigo

Figure 4.4: The set up for a simple cool caloric test. The patient (the author in this case) has a waterproof apron around his neck and is holding a kidney dish to catch the irrigating water. The head of the couch is raised to lie at an angle of about 30° with the horizontal.

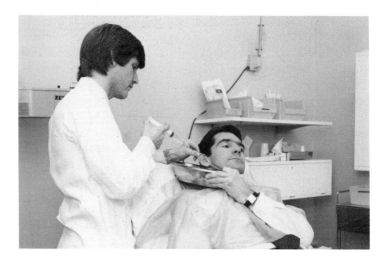

and vomiting, but simply to detect whether the labyrinth is functioning. Ice-cold water has been suggested as the stimulus, and whilst it certainly induces a brisk response the cold water itself induces a very unpleasant sensation and is better not used as water at 20 or 25°C (68 or 77°F) is adequate. The reaction is dependent solely on the temperature of the water and not the degree of force used to irrigate the ear canal. It is quite enough to trickle the water in over a period of 20 seconds. Do this with a 20 ml syringe attached to a soft flexible tip — a Kwill or a large plastic Medicut or similar intravenous cannula is suitable. Put the tip of the cannula only a very little way into the ear canal and aim the stream of water at the roof of the canal (Figure 4.5). When you have used up the water in the syringe, ask the patient to stare at a point on the ceiling whilst you watch their eyes. Nystagmus may well develop and the fast phase will be away from the ear you have just irrigated. Ask the patient what they feel and whether the sensation you have just

Figure 4.5: A close up view of the irrigation procedure for a cool caloric. Here a small metal cannula has been used to run the water along the roof of the canal, but a small plastic cannula does just as well. The tip of the cannula is pointed at the roof of the canal and the water run in gently. Twenty ml of water is usually adequate to induce an obvious response.

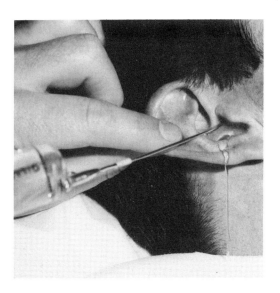

produced is the same as their complaint. This often helps to confirm or deny that vertigo, rather than some other form of dizziness, is their problem. If you have any Frenzel's glasses, put them on the patient as the nystagmus is fading away, switch on the little built-in illuminators and switch off the room light. In a normal ear, or one with a labyrinthine disorder the nystagmus is enhanced whilst in a central disorder there is usually no change.

Wait for the nystagmus to settle, give the patient five minutes' rest and repeat the test using the same volume, same temperature and same duration of irrigation on the other side. Although this test cannot be quantitative you may get some idea of the relative condition of the two sides by starting a stopwatch as you begin the irrigation and using as an end-point the moment the nystagmus stops whilst the patient is fixating on some point of the ceiling.

Do not be alarmed if you fail to get a response on both sides as this can occur physiologically in ballet dancers, ice-skaters (Dix and Hood 1969), divers and even aircraft pilots (Coles and Knight 1961) who have developed the ability to suppress labyrinthine function provided vision is intact and the eyes are open. An absent response on one side is called a canal paresis and indicates loss or diminution of function of the vestibular labyrinth, nerve or nuclei on that side. Paresis is not really a very good term for the failure of a sensory structure but it has become firmly entrenched in the literature and is unlikely to be changed.

Bithermal calorics

An imbalance between the two sides of the vestibular system whether it be caused by disease or be part of the normal differences that can occur between right and left, can affect the caloric test. The nystagmus induced by the test may be enhanced in one or other direction and this feature is called 'directional preponderance'. It can confuse a single temperature caloric test, apparently masking or making worse a canal paresis. To overcome this problem bithermal caloric tests were introduced by Fitzgerald and Hallpike (1942) and have remained the standard procedure for evaluating vestibular function. This test requires slightly more sophisticated apparatus as the ears have to be irrigated with water at 30°C and 44°C, i.e. 7°C above and below body temperature. The position of the patient is the same as in the cool caloric but you need two tanks of water at the required temperature. The water should be run through a cannula into the ear canal for 40 s and a total of about 250 ml of water be used. This is easily achieved by having the tanks on a shelf about 4 feet above the level of the couch, with some tubing siphoning the water off. A 14 G cannula on the end of the tubing gives a flow rate of about 400 ml/min and a pair of artery forceps clamped on the tube can be released to start the flow and reapplied at the end of 40 seconds. The beginning of the irrigation is taken as time zero and, using a stop-watch, the end-point is recorded as the time at which the nystagmus ceases when the patient is fixing hard at some point on the ceiling (Figure 4.6). A small mark on the ceiling positioned so that the eyes are looking straight ahead is useful for this. If you have Frenzel's glasses these can be put in place at

Figure 4.6: A simple arrangement for performing the bithermal caloric test. The nurse has a clamp on the tubing which siphons water from the 30° tank. She starts a stop-watch at the beginning of the irrigation and when 40 seconds have passed reapplies the clamp, but leaves the stop-watch running so that the duration of the induced nystagmus can be timed. At the end of the irrigation the patient turns his head back to the central positon and stares at a mark on the ceiling whilst the nystagmus is timed.

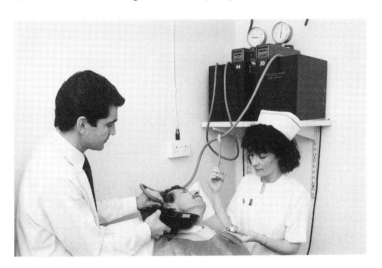

the end-point of the nystagmus to see if loss of fixation results in the reappearance of nystagmus.

The sequence is to perform 30°C left, 30°C right, 44°C left, 44°C right and to note the duration of the nystagmus for each of the four irrigations. The results can be plotted on a standard form (Figure 4.7). The combination of a canal paresis and a directional preponderance can be difficult to assess from these sorts of charts but a simple calculation helps separate the two effects. Using the duration of the nystagmus in seconds, then:

$$\text{a. canal paresis} = \frac{(L30 + L44) - (R30 + R44)}{(L30 + L44) + (R30 + R44)} \times 100\%$$

a +ve value indicates a right canal paresis: a −ve value indicates a left canal paresis.

Figure 4.7: A typical record chart for bithermal calorics showing a normal response. The irrigation is performed for 40 s and the end-point of the duration of the nystagmus marked for each temperature and ear by the arrows above each of the four tracings. The duration of the nystagmus is slightly less for the warm (44°C) irrigation, and this is a normal finding. Various combinations indicate a canal paresis, directional preponderance or some combination and are best evaluated by use of the formulae given in the text.

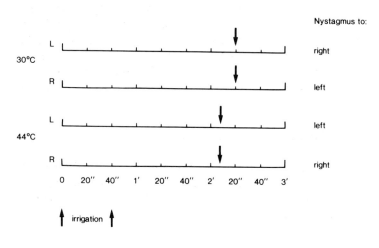

Normal Bithermal Caloric Test

There is quite a wide range of responses in normal subjects tested with visual fixation and a figure of more than 20–25% should be obtained from the test to indicate any degree of canal paresis.

The directional preponderance (DD) can also be calculated by the relationship:

$$\text{b. directional preponderance} = \frac{(L30 + R44) - (L44 + R30)}{(L30 + R44) + (R30 + R44)} \times 100\%$$

a +ve value indicates directional preponderance of the nystagmus to the right; a −ve value indicates directional preponderance of the nystagmus to the left.

The value of calculating the directional preponderance is probably limited as it can originate from many parts of the vestibular system both central and peripheral, but the reason for performing bithermal calorics is to eliminate this effect so that the degree of 'paralysis' of the right or left vestibular labyrinth, nerve or nuclei can be assessed. A bilateral partial paralysis is more difficult to assess but in the normal subject the duration of the nystagmus has a range of from 90 to 135 seconds with the hot response often being a little shorter than the cold response (Hood and Korres 1979). Knowing these values can help decide whether a bilateral canal weakness or even hypersensitivity is present.

There are many difficulties with interpreting caloric test results as the stimulus to the labyrinth is not physiological and cannot be accurately controlled. It has been likened to trying to test the knee-jerk with a sledge hammer but in spite of the difficulties bithermal caloric testing remains the cornerstone of vestibular testing.

OTHER FORMS OF NYSTAGMUS

Various other types of nystagmus occur as do several forms of irregular eye movement. Many are not associated with dizziness but may suggest that there is some underlying defect with vision or other parts of the brain.

Congenital nystagmus

Congenital nystagmus may be familial, and although often not recognised at birth persists throughout life without symptoms although it often causes discomfort in anyone talking to the owner. Several forms of eye movement occur, with both eyes being equally affected. There can be purely pendular nystagmus with the amplitude of the oscillations varying from minute to minute and with the direction of gaze. Exaggerated irregular vestibular-type nystagmus with crazy jerking of the eyes may be present but frequently there is some contribution from the two types, making description difficult. There is usually one direction of gaze in which the nystagmus is minimal, and the head is usually moved so that the eyes are in this position during fixation, as visual activity tends to diminish with increasing nystagmus. Surprisingly, eye closure virtually always abolishes the erratic movements in nearly all cases (Forssmann 1964) but abolishing fixation in darkness or with Frenzel's glasses has an unpredictable effect.

Congenital nystagmus as described is idiopathic but other forms of nystagmus, especially the pendular variety can be secondary to visual defects or acquired disorders.

Ocular nystagmus

Congenital blindness, either from disorders of the eye as in albinism, aniridia, opacities, and so on, or from central disorders, upsets the acquisition of the ability to fixate and commonly results in a pendular nystagmus. Acquired blindness can also produce this pendular form. As in the congenital nystagmus group, balance is not affected, and dizziness does not result, diagnosis being easily made.

Latent nystagmus

This peculiar form of nystagmus can also fall into the group of ocular nystagmus and it is usually associated with a squint or poor vision in one or both eyes from childhood.

At rest with the eyes open there is nothing abnormal to be seen, but when one eye is covered a vestibular type horizontal nystagmus towards the uncovered eye develops in both eyes. The nystagmus changes direction when the cover is removed from the first eye and placed on the other. During the nystagmus the visual acuity falls.

The reason for describing these forms of nystagmus is that the dizziness can arise as an independent occurrence and the presence of nystagmus can cause confusion and add to the difficulties in diagnosis.

Acquired pendular nystagmus

Pure pendular nystagmus, where there is no difference in the speed of the two components, can arise from disease in the brain. Multiple sclerosis appears to be the commonest cause (Aschoff, Conrad and Kornhuber 1974), but it may also arise in strokes, vascular malformations and following encephalitis. The eye movements are frequently horizontal but may be vertical in a quarter of the multiple sclerosis cases. The eye movements can be binocular or monocular with the eyes moving in synchrony or not. Unlike the congenital pendular nystagmus in the acquired form, there is no particular position of gaze in which the nystagmus is minimal. Another important distinction is that these patients almost always have oscillopsia, that is a complaint of the surroundings bobbing up and down or swinging from side to side, depending upon the direction of the nystagmus, and this may make them unsteady when they are moving around.

DISORDERS OF EYE MOVEMENT IN CEREBELLAR DISEASE

The cerebellum is involved in the co-ordination of eye movements and disorders can result not only in spontaneous nystagmus but also in failure to perform voluntary eye movements. Some of the patterns of eye movement that arise are quite peculiar and are sometimes given the name of 'ataxic nystagmus' which is really a contradiction in terms as something without order (ataxia) cannot really be rhythmic and oscillating.

In acute central cerebellar disease the truncal ataxia that occurs is also expressed in eye movements where gross jerks of large amplitude in all directions of gaze occur, the movement in one eye often being unrelated to that in the other. Another peculiarity termed macro-saccadic oscillations may arise where both eyes move together in short bursts of very rapid, large, but equal, amplitude, horizontal to and fro excursions that occur on changing the direction of gaze. Should the patient survive the onslaught of the disease this 'nystagmus' frequently fades away.

In acute disease of the cerebellar hemispheres a rather coarse nystagmus of large amplitude, but of a slower speed than typical vestibular nystagmus, may appear. It is easier to see than a vestibular nystagmus and is usually found with the patient looking to the side of the lesion.

Longstanding generalised cerebellar disease may result in two further sorts of nystagmus, one of which may come our way because of associated unsteadiness.

Isolated down beat nystagmus is a nystagmus with a fast phase beating downwards that occurs on gaze straight ahead. Looking up or down makes it disappear but, surprisingly, looking a little to each side in the same horizontal plane enhances it. All the patients tend to have bobbing oscillopsia even at rest and this is frequently their presenting complaint.

A separate phenomenon is called rebound nystagmus. Here a typical horizontal vestibular-type nystagmus is present in one direction of gaze. It is first degree, with the fast phase beating in the same direction. It dies away after ten to thirty seconds but when the eyes return to the central position a horizontal vestibular nystagmus in the opposite direction appears and persists for a shorter time than the first degree nystagmus.

Voluntary eye movements may also be affected and make their appearance as the inability to follow a slowly moving target smoothly. What occurs is a jerky movement when the patient is moving the eyes in the direction of the side of the lesion. This is a simple test to perform. Ask the patient to look at the tip of your finger that you are holding out at about his arm's-length in front of his face. Now move your hand slowly to one side then the other. You should take two or three seconds to get to each side from the central position. In bilateral cerebellar disease the jerky movements are present in both directions. The next thing to test for is the inability to fix accurately on a target. Overshoot commonly occurs and the eyes have to make a second, third or even fourth small movement to home in on the target. This is best tested by having the patient look at the tip of the finger of one of your hands held in front of his face and then change the direction of his gaze to a finger of your other hand, held to one side.

Although the description of these various tests of eye movement takes a while to describe they are quick to perform and after a while can be built in to the rest of the examination so that you develop a smooth procedure that includes everything you want to test.

STANCE, GAIT AND CO-ORDINATION

Watching the patient enter the room and walk to the chair often provides some clues to their disability. Several features are common to nearly all patients with a disorder of balance and dizziness. They are usually unhappy to move their head quickly and so make slow deliberate movements with apparently a stiff neck. They often walk with the feet spaced wider than seems normal and may move from one support to next. Acute labyrinthine or cerebellar lesions tend to push the patient to the same side as the disease, so they might have a tendency to veer off to one side. In cerebellar disease the head tends to be held a little to the affected side and the arm on that side lies still against the side of the body and does not swing in time with the legs. Observations specific to particular conditions are described later in the appropriate sections, but the patient with hysteria provides a parody of unsteadiness, making extreme movements (which actually tests their balance mechanisms to the full) yet rarely falling.

After you have taken the history, stressing the patient's ability to balance and co-ordinate with simple tests, may help illuminate the site of the trouble.

Romberg's test

Generations of medical students have floundered on the question 'What is Romberg's test?' or 'What does Romberg's sign mean?'. A description of the original test, its significance and subsequent corruption is given in detail by Rogers (1980), whereas Edwards (1973) gives probably the best description of how to perform the test. In essence the patient is asked to stand unsupported, with feet together side by side, and then to close his eyes, when any effect on his stance is noted. Now, anyone

55

without explanation and reassurance that you are not going to let them fall is quite likely to sway if you order them to suddenly close their eyes. This is especially true if they are standing far from any support and their complaint is dizziness. So to perform the test, have the patient standing with a chair behind them. Whilst you stand in front with arms outstretched each side of them, but not touching (Figure 4.8). Tell them what you are going to do and that they will not fall.

Start off with their feet apart and ask them to close their eyes for three or four seconds. See what happens and if there is only slight unsteadiness make them bring their feet closer together and repeat the procedure if possible, until their feet are side by side. The eyes need only be closed for a few seconds. A normal person may sway very slightly with eyes open and perhaps a little more with them closed. Romberg's test was originally applied to syphilitics where disease in the posterior columns of the spinal cord cut off somatosensory information from the legs. Balance in these people was therefore normally maintained by vision and the vestibular labyrinth providing for the loss of somatosenory information from the legs when standing. Closing the eyes removed this protective effect and so the patient swayed from side to side with increasing amplitude and would eventually fall as the labyrinth is incapable of maintaining posture on its own. The same finding arises in other diseases that affect the somatosensors and this is a positive Romberg's test.

Subsequently, the interpretation of the outcome of this test has been extended in an attempt to aid assessment of laby-rinthine or central disease. A synopsis of the interpretation of the test results is given in Table 4.5. Apart from the changes with the somatosensory loss, the guidelines should not be applied too strictly, and of course if the patient cannot stand unaided Romberg's test is quite useless.

Gait

Asking the patient to walk in a straight line first of all with the eyes open and then with the eyes closed provides a more severe test of balance. The patient need only walk four or five metres across the room as this gives long enough to assess them and allows an assistant to be close enough to give them moral, if not

Figure 4.8: Romberg's test.
(a) Start off with the feet apart, and having reassured the patient they are not going to be allowed to fall, ask them to close their eyes and count slowly to four. If there is no major increase in the amount of sway with the eyes closed then the test is repeated with the feet brought closer together until finally (b) the procedure is performed with the feet together.

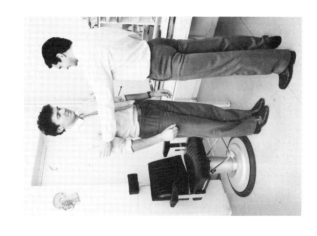

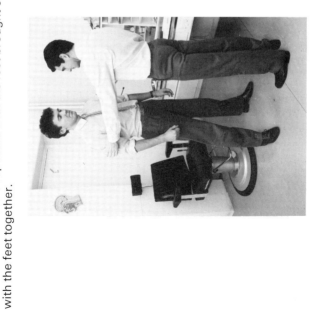

Table 4.5: Romberg's test

	Eyes open	Eyes closed
Normal	Steady	Steady or slight sway
Disease		
(a) Somatosensory loss	Steady	Unsteady — falls
(b) Central lesion i.e. cerebellar	Unsteady (tends to fall to same side)	Unsteady No change — may even improve
(c) Labyrinthine		
1. Unilateral chronic compensated	Steady	Slight sway
2. Bilateral complete loss — compensated	Steady	Unsteady — falls
3. Acute	Unsteady (tends to fall to same side)	Worse (tends to fall to same side)
(d) Hysteria	Steady/Unsteady	Worse, exaggerated Topples — but usually recovers

actual support. Table 4.6 gives a breakdown of the likely outcomes. Of course there are many modifications of the tests of stance and gait that by making the procedure more demanding sometimes shed a brighter light on the underlying condition. Fregly (1974) has modified Romberg's test by having the patient hold his arms across his chest and stand heel to toe, and Fukuda (1959) has developed a test whereby the patient walks on the spot with eyes closed and the angular deviation from his original position is measured. The original articles give all the details.

Co-ordination

In this part of the examination we are looking for ataxia. As defined in Chapter 2, muscle weakness or joint stiffness from whatever cause should have been excluded as this will in itself result in some inco-ordination. Major changes in visual acuity will probably have been recognised by the patient and this leaves us with labyrinthine, somatosensory and cerebellar disease to untangle. The procedures described here are designed to sort out cerebellar defects.

The symptoms of acute midline cerebellar disease are

Table 4.6: Straight line walking

	Eyes open	Eyes closed
Normal	No deviation	No or slight deviation
Disease		
(a) Somatosensory loss	No deviation	Great difficulty — very unsteady
(b) Central	Variety of effects	Variety of effects
Cerebellar	Veers to diseased side	Less severe
(c) Labyrinthine		
1. Unilateral chronic compensated	No deviation, or may veer to side	Worse
2. Bilateral chronic compensated	No deviation	Worse — may be impossible because of unsteadiness
3. Acute	Veers to side of lesion	Impossible
(d) Hysteria	Frequent deviation both sides	Wild deviations — but does not fall

frequently severe and disabling with truncal ataxia causing gross, sometimes disastrous, unsteadiness and vertigo whenever the patient moves from rest. However, if the body is supported, arm and hand movements are usually intact and normal. With lateral cerebellar disease ataxia of the arms and legs of the same side of the body makes its appearance, the extent depending on both the severity and speed of onset of the defect. The gait is altered with gross disease but lesser degrees of derangement produce changes in the control of muscle tone and movement, limited to one side. Many tests have been devised to elicit limb ataxia and fall into three groups which depend on the ability:

1. to perform rapid fine movements accurately;
2. to exchange smoothly from one motor function to another, exactly the opposite (diadochokinesia);
3. to co-ordinate the movement of the whole arm or leg accurately.

A reasonable test sequence is as follows.

Ask the patient to touch the tip of first index, then the middle, ring and little fingers with the tip of the thumb of the same hand, and then return from little to ring to middle and index and keep repeating the procedure (Figure 4.9). You may need to show them how to perform this by doing it yourself.

Figure 4.9: Test of the ability to perform fine movements. The tip of the thumb is moved from finger to finger so that the contact is made in the order index, middle, ring and little, then back again.

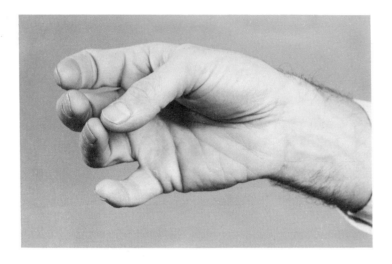

Ask them to perform the same test with the other hand. There are usually some slight differences from right to left, depending on the handedness of the individual but they are rarely marked. Cerebellar disease may cause obvious slowness and defects in accuracy of placement.

Now, ask them to place the palm of one hand comfortably on the front of the forearm of the other side. They then have to turn the hand over so that the back of it rests on the forearm, and when this is done, return to the original position, and then keep repeating the procedure quickly, but not to try to achieve a world record for speed. Test one side then the other. A clumsy flailing of the arm on one side is called dysdiadochokinesis (Figure 4.10).

Finally, ask the patient to touch the tip of his nose with the index finger of one of his hands. Then hold up your index finger in front of his face at a bit less than the patient's arm's-length away (Figure 4.11). Now, ask him to move from the tip of his nose to touch the tip of your index finger, and then return his finger back to the tip of his nose. Repeat this a few times until they have got the idea then slowly move your hand 20 or

Figure 4.10: One way of testing for dysdiadochokinesis. The palm of one hand is placed on the opposite forearm and then is turned over so that the back of the hand rests on the forearm. After turning back again the procedure is repeated rapidly several times.

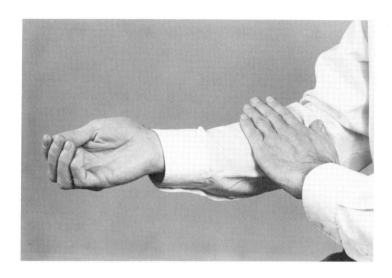

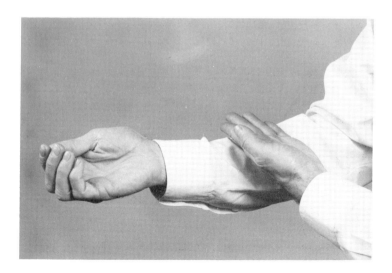

Figure 4.11: Positioning for the finger–nose test. After getting the idea of the procedure the examiner moves his hand slowly from side to side whilst the patient continues touching the tip of her nose then the examiner's index finger. This gives the examiner the chance to watch eye movements during slow pursuit.

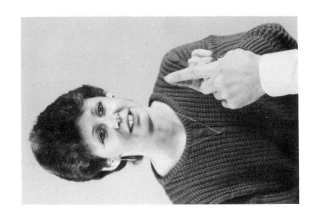

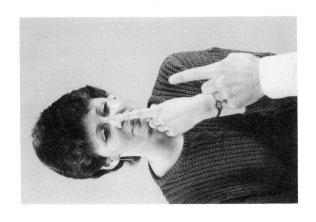

30 cm to one side then the other whilst they continue to touch their nose and your fingertip. Doing this also gives you a chance to watch the eye movements. After a few traverses stop back at the midline.

Many patients will have some form of tremor, and this will affect their performance in the test but patients with cerebellar disorders will overshoot the target, usually to the same side and have much more difficulty with the moving target. The static part of this finger–nose test should now be done with the patient closing his eyes after a few trial runs to establish the position of your index finger in his mind's eye. With cerebellar lesions there is no real change but in somatosensory disorders of the arm or shoulder a normal or near normal performance will disintegrate with eye closure, the searching finger only finding its target after random movement.

The same effect occurs with eye closure in the preceding two tests; in cerebellar disease little change, in somatosensory disorders ataxia arises in the dark.

Similar tests can be devised to test the legs. Rapid plantar- then dorsiflexion of the raised foot, tests for diadochokinesis whilst moving the heel of one foot from knee to ankle along the inside of the calf of the other leg tests co-ordination of the whole leg, and is called the heel–shin test in later chapters.

THE CRANIAL NERVES

This is not the place to describe the detailed examination of the cranial nerves but some features are more important in the dizzy patient and these will be described.

Optic nerve and fundi (II)

Visual acuity can be estimated by the ability to perceive light, count fingers and read decreasing sizes of print. The visual fields can be simply tested one eye at a time by confrontation, asking the patient when they can see your moving fingertip as it is brought from behind to in front of their head from various directions (Figure 4.12).

The ophthalmoscope is an invaluable instrument provided you continue to use it regularly. Opacities in the lens and the

Figure 4.12: Simple testing of the visual field. The examiner sits at about arm's-length from the patient. The eyes are covered as shown and the examiner's hand is brought forward from behind the patient's head. The examiner's index finger is moved a little and the patient, who should be looking directly at the examiner's eye, is asked to respond when he can see the moving finger. Repeating the procedure from different directions gives an indication of the extent of the visual fields and can detect major losses.

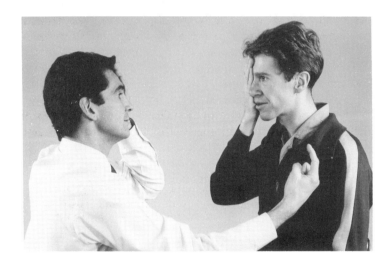

two chambers can be detected, and if not severe, direct inspection of the retina and optic nerve head can be performed. Degenerative vascular disease, diabetes and papilloedema are amongst the many conditions that may make their appearance alter and which are of interest to us. Several beautiful colour atlases of retinoscopy are now published and are worth study if only to be able to recognise the common conditions.

Oculomotor, trochlear, abducent (III, IV, VI)

The ophthalmoscope can also be used as a source of light to test the pupillary reflexes. Do not shine the light directly into the eye from the front, rather from an angle, and watch for constriction not only of the pupil of the eye you are testing but also the other eye. Test both eyes, then ask the patient to gaze at a distant object for a few seconds and then try to look at the tip of his own nose whilst you look for the normal pupillary constriction that accompanies accommodation when focusing on a near target. These pupillary responses are brought about by the IIIrd nerve. Eye movements are finally mediated by the muscles supplied by nerves III, IV and VI, and the directions in which these muscles pull are shown in Figure 4.13. These are tested by asking the patient, whose head should stay still, to follow your finger in the eight directions, and watching for limitation of movement whilst asking if they have any double vision, suggesting a weakness of one set of muscles that may not be visible to you.

The trigeminal (V)

When a nerve is being stretched, pulled or compressed loss of the sensory component of a mixed motor and sensory nerve

Figure 4.13: Directions of movement of the right eye in response to the pull of the six extraocular muscles. The two oblique muscles and the superior and inferior recti cause not only a major deviation in the direction shown but also a little rotation.

DIRECTIONS OF EYE MOVEMENT

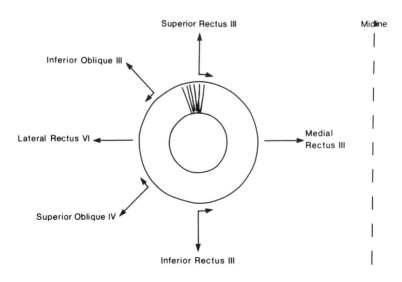

65

tends to occur first. Loss of sensation in the distribution of the
Vth nerve is therefore an important sign to elicit, as growths in
the cerebello-pontine angle may affect the nerve. The cutaneous
distribution is shown in Figure 4.14. Remember that the skin
over the angle of the jaw is supplied by the greater auricular
nerve from cervical roots 2 and 3 and that C1 has no cutaneous
distribution. Loss of light touch sensation is likely to be lost
before pain, so testing with a wisp of cotton wool is probably
best. Ask the patient to close his eyes and tell you when he feels
a light touch with the cotton wool. The cornea, which has a
sensory supply from the ophthalmic division of V, is by far the
most sensitive part to test. Pull out a wisp of cotton wool and
ask the patient to look slightly to the right whilst you test the left
eye. From the side, gently draw the strands of cotton wool
across the edge of the cornea which extends from the outer

Figure 4.14: Approximate distribution of the cutaneous
sensation of the head and neck. There is often overlap and
variation in the distribution especially of the branches of the
cervical roots.

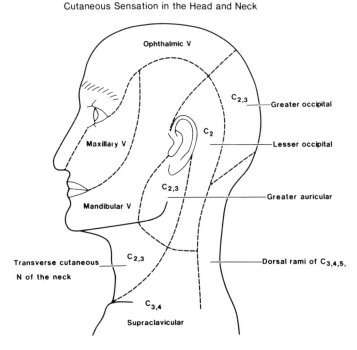

Cutaneous Sensation in the Head and Neck

perimeter of the iris and covers the pupil (Figure 4.15). There may be a reflex lid closure in both eyes, then test the right side with the patient looking to the left. Again, look for the blink reflex and ask if the sensation is the same on both sides. The blink reflex is still useful even in a one-side facial palsy.

Facial (VII)

Damage to the facial nerve below its nucleus in the brainstem (a lower motor neurone lesion) results in weakness of the same side of the face. This can be complete or partial with different portions of the face being spared or involved. With a complete loss there is asymmetry of the face which remains motionless on the affected side. The eyebrow droops, the lines on the forehead and the nasolabial fold are smoothed out. The eyelids may be wider apart because the elevators of the upper lid (supplied by III) are continuing to act. Efforts to close the eye cause the eyeball to roll upwards and the lids fail to move so that if there is residual function in the lacrimal glands tears well up as they

Figure 4.15: Testing the corneal reflex. A wisp of cotton wool is touched lightly against the cornea. There is a blink which indicates an intact corneal reflex. If there is a facial palsy on the tested side then the blink can be seen in the other eye.

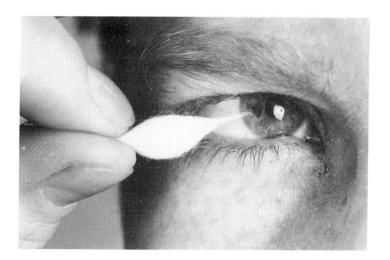

are not swept towards the opening of the lacrimal sac which in any case may not be making contact with the conjunctiva. The nostrils do not move on breathing, and when a smile is attempted the lips are drawn up on the unaffected side. On trying to whistle, the lips fail to pucker up. During eating, food tends to accumulate on the affected side through paralysis of buccinator and the patient may dribble.

The same constellation of signs occurs in damage to the facial nerve nucleus but a supranuclear (upper motor neurone) lesion results in a different distribution of loss. The part of the facial nucleus that supplies the facial muscles above the eye is supplied by both cerebral hemispheres, whilst the rest of the nucleus is supplied only by the contralateral hemisphere (Figure 4.16). A stroke involving one cerebral hemisphere can result in the patient being able to frown and close his eyes, whilst being quite unable to move his lips on the same side. A further peculiarity that may occur is the dissociation between voluntary and emotional responses. When asked to show his teeth, he cannot but will smile normally in response to something funny.

Other branches of the facial nerve supply structures whose loss of function may not be noticed. The chorda tympani delivers taste sensation from the front two-thirds of the tongue, whilst the nerve to stapedius supplies the small muscle that attaches to the stapes. Loss of this latter function is only very occasionally noticed as increased hearing on that side (hyperacusis), whilst loss of taste is frequently insignificant compared to the gross facial deformity. The facial nerve also supplies the secretory fibres to the lacrimal glands, the submandibular and sublingual salivary glands and makes contributions to the parotid. Reduction in the output is rarely noticed. However, all three functions, taste, stapedius muscle activity and the production of tears can be tested.

Lacrimation

Use two strips of blotting paper 5 mm wide and 50 mm long bent over at one end for a distance of 5 mm. Carefully hang one strip over each lower lid by the short limb of the strip. This is not painful and is sufficient to induce lacrimation. Using smelling salts to make the eyes water may serve to confuse the results. Wait 5 minutes then remove both strips and mark the excursion of the tears and measure the distance in mm from the bend. Tearing is abnormal in one eye when the difference in the

Figure 4.16: Innervation of the left VIIN nucleus. Most of the 'voluntary' innervation of the nucleus of the left VIIN comes from opposite cerebral hemisphere. However, some comes from the hemisphere of the same side and this contribution supplies that part of the nucleus involved with movement of the eyes and forehead. This accounts for the sparing of the eyes and the forehead following a 'stroke' — an upper motor neurone lesion.

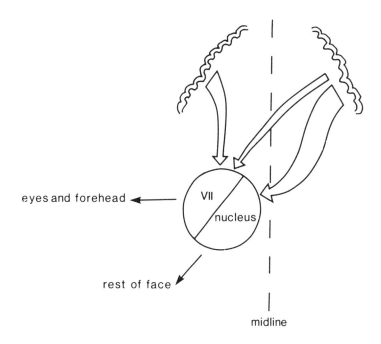

lengths is more than 30% of the total length of both, i.e. ((good − bad)/(good + bad)) × 100. Tearing is deficient in both eyes when the total length of both sides is less than 25 mm (Figure 4.17).

Taste

This can be tested with cotton buds dipped in solutions of sugar, salt and vinegar but this is a qualitative procedure and a reliable quantitative procedure is yet to be developed. Using an electrical current to stimulate the taste fibres can give some indication of differences between the two sides but changes have not been found to correlate well with the degree of degeneration in the nerve — unlike the tests of lacrimation.

Figure 4.17: Schirmer's test. The individual here has a right sided facial palsy and poor lacrimation on that side. The extent of excursion of the tears is indicated by the stippling.

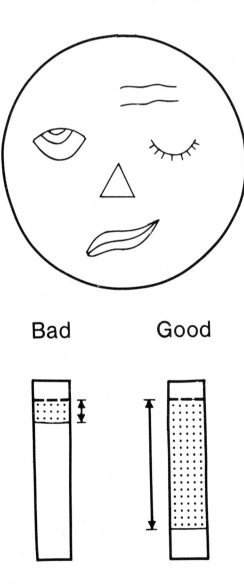

Stapedial reflexes

Testing the action of the stapedius muscle is really quite simple but requires the use of a tympanometer and this will be described in the glossary on auditory testing.

Acoustic and vestibular nerves (VIII)

This section deals with testing the hearing. For practical purposes the ear is divided into three portions; outer, middle and inner. The outer portion comprises the auricle and ear canal. The middle ear consists of the eardrum with a chain of three small bones, malleus, incus and stapes, linking the eardrum to the inner ear. This mechanism serves to collect the vibrations of air-borne sound and convert them into pressure changes within the inner ear. The cochlear portion of the inner ear converts the pressure changes from the incoming sound into nerve impulses which are subsequently perceived as speech, music or some other noisy feature of our daily life. Loss of hearing can arise because sound is not conducted to the inner ear — a conductive deafness — or because the cochlea or the nerve are not working — a sensorineural deafness (Figure 4.18). Sometimes the hearing loss will be mixed, with both a conductive and sensorineural component, being present. With easy clinical tests it is possible to distinguish between these two forms of deafness and also get a rough idea of the level of hearing loss. More sophisticated equipment is needed to distinguish between a cochlear and a neural deafness and a section on audiometry is included in the glossary at the end of the book.

The whisper test

First you have to assess the general level of hearing in each ear. Tell the patient that you are going to whisper in one ear at a time and as soon as he hears what you say to repeat the word out loud. Sit on one side of the patient so that he cannot see your lips and stretch out one arm behind his head with one of your fingers resting on the tragus (the triangular piece of cartilage in front of the ear canal of the non-test ear). Gently rub or move this to produce masking noise in the non-test ear, then, softly whisper a word into the ear now facing you (Figure 4.19). Properly done, you should use two syllable words (spondees) with equal stress on each syllable. Words such as birthday, arm-

Figure 4.18: Diagram to illustrate the possible sites of hearing loss. Deafness can be conductive secondary to disease in the ear canal and middle ear, or sensorineural (sometimes called perceptive). Sensorineural deafness can be further split into cochlear (sensory) or neural depending on the site of the lesion.

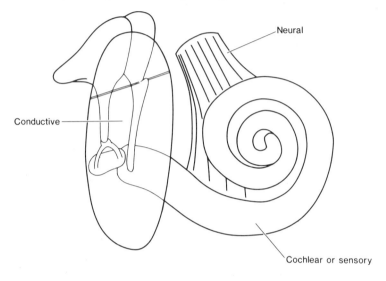

Figure 4.19: Demonstration of whisper test. The patient is turned so that she is unable to see the examiner's lips, and a masking noise is made in the non-test ear by gently rubbing the tragus.

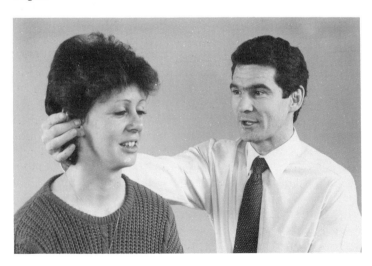

chair, doormat, duckpond and so on can be used, tailoring the words for the very young patient. If they cannot repeat the soft whispers, repeat the word more loudly each time until they get it correct. You may have to have a few trial runs with children until they get the idea of what to do, but eventually you should end up with a rough appraisal of whether they can hear a soft whisper (normal), loud whisper (about 20–30 dB hearing level), a softly spoken voice (30–40 dB), a normally spoken voice (40–50 dB) or a loudly spoken voice (more than 50 dB). The dB figures are only a very rough guide to the average hearing loss.

When one ear has been tested change sides and repeat the procedure.

Next, you need a tuning fork. The low frequency forks — 128 Hz and 256 Hz — are not really suitable as they can give an unreliable response by stimulating the vibration sensors; use a 512 Hz tuning fork instead.

Weber test

Explain that you are going to put the base of the tuning fork on the patient's forehead and if they hear it they should point to whether they hear it in the middle or in one ear. Do not whack the tuning fork on the edge of your desk, it is quite enough to use the base of your thumb, knee or elbow. If they cannot hear anything even when you have hit the tuning fork a bit harder, try placing the base of the fork on the upper incisor teeth, this seems to make the test more sensitive — unless they have dentures (Figure 4.20).

In a conductive deafness, the tuning fork is heard in the deaf ear, whilst in a sensorineural deafness it is heard in the good ear. If the hearing is normal or symmetrically poor then the sound of the tuning fork will probably be heard in the middle (Figure 4.21). Since you already know the approximate level of the hearing from the whisper test, the results of the Weber test start to suggest whether any unilateral loss is conductive or sensorineural. Various combinations can, of course, confuse this simple pattern so then we go on to the Rinne test to sort out the more difficult problems or to confirm the simple ones.

The Rinne test

The Rinne test relies on the principle that in the normal ear a vibrating tuning fork is heard better when held in the air near

Figure 4.20: The Weber test. The foot of the tuning fork is placed on the forehead in the midline and the patient asked to indicate where sound is heard. The patient's eyes often move to the side on which the sound is heard and this is sometimes helpful.

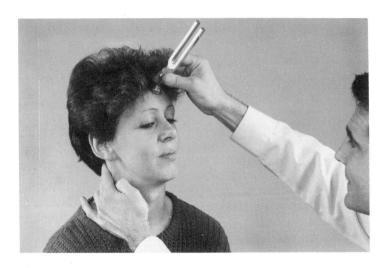

Figure 4.21: The Weber test. Here the direction of deviation of the eyes indicates the side on which the tuning fork is heard. The Weber is heard in the deaf ear in a unilateral conductive deafness and in the good ear in a unilateral sensorineural deafness.

WEBER TEST

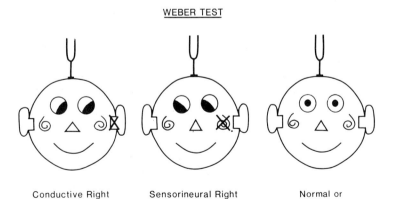

Conductive Right   Sensorineural Right   Normal or
Symmetrical Loss

the ear canal than when the foot of the fork is placed on the bony mastoid prominence behind the ear. In a moderate conductive hearing loss the reverse is true with the bone conduction (BC) being better than the air conduction (AC). This is called a Rinne negative result, the normal ear being Rinne positive. The exact mechanism of this is unclear and need not bother us. In a unilateral sensorineural loss the result in the deaf ear should be Rinne positive (AC>BC), but now the presence of the other ear starts to interfere. When the tuning fork is on the mastoid the vibrations are transmitted via the skull to the other ear and are heard there with only slight loss of intensity. What therefore happens is that the air conduction is poor because little sound is heard transmitted through the air to the other ear, whilst bone conduction is apparently good giving a negative Rinne that falsely indicates a conductive loss. The way to overcome this false negative result is to create a masking noise in the non-test ear, much as we did for the whisper test, and repeat the Rinne test when the correct positive result is obtained (Figure 4.22).

There are several ways to perform the Rinne test but I will describe the modified Rinne where you ask the patient to compare the loudness of air conduction to bone conduction. Explain that you are going to hold the tuning fork in front of the ear and then on the bone behind the ear and that you want them to tell you which sound is louder. Set the tuning fork vibrating gently and hold it so that its tip is about 1 cm from the ear canal. Hold the fork so that the wide surface of one of the blades is facing the ear. Say this is the front one or first sound, let them appreciate the level for a few seconds then transfer the fork and place the foot firmly on the mastoid. After a few seconds say this is the back one or second sound and ask which was louder, front or back, first or second. Take care not to touch the prongs whilst transferring the fork. If the test is negative and you suspect it might be a false negative because of the findings from whispering and from the Weber test then ask the patient to wiggle the tragus of the other ear with his finger whilst you repeat the test or carry out the masking procedure yourself as in the whispering test (Figure 4.23).

A flow chart for the case of a unilateral hearing loss is shown in Table 4.7. A true Rinne negative result in a conductive deafness suggests that the loss is more than 30 dB, whereas a positive result suggests that it is less than this. Unfortunately, a

Figure 4.22: Rinne test finding. In the normal ear the air-borne sound is heard better than that transmitted by way of the mastoid bone. The reverse is true for a moderate conductive loss. Confusion sometimes arises with a sensorineural loss when the good ear hears the bone conduction thereby giving a false result. This is overcome by introducing a masking noise in the good, non-test ear.

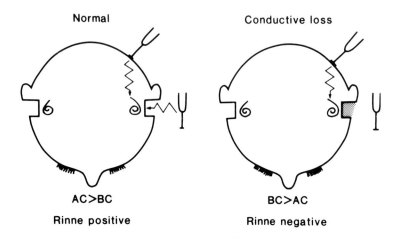

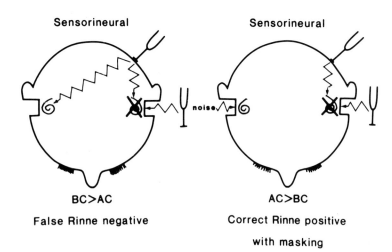

Figure 4.23: The Rinne test.
(a) Shows the correct way of holding the tuning fork for air conduction.
(b) Shows the foot of the tuning fork placed on the mastoid, while a masking noise is made in the opposite ear.

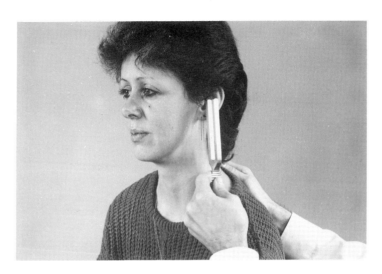

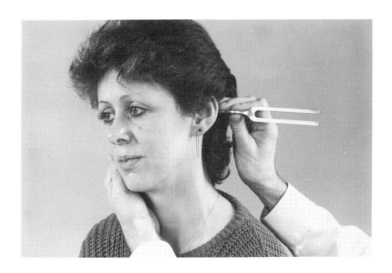

Table 4.7: Scheme for assessing unilateral hearing test

	Whisper Test	
	Reduced hearing in one ear	
	Weber Test	
Lateralises to bad side		Lateralises to good side
Conductive		Sensorineural
	Rinne Test	
Rinne positive	Rinne negative	False Rinne negative
Mild conductive	Moderate conductive	Repeat with masking
or sensorineural		Rinne positive
		Sensorineural

number of individuals fail to convert to a Rinne negative result until a greater difference between air and bone conduction occurs. The Rinne positive result is therefore not a firm indicator of the lack of moderate conductive loss, whilst a Rinne negative result does give a good indication of a moderate or severe conductive loss. Bilateral sensorineural or conductive losses may give equivocal Weber results but can usually be assessed on the combination of the whisper tests and Rinne tests. A combination of a sensorineural loss in one ear and conductive loss in the other is probably the most difficult to sort out, even for the experts. If the non-test ear is the one with the conductive loss it might be impossible to get enough masking noise in to overcome the false negative Rinne in the test ear. In practice, a conductive loss is very frequently associated with visible pathology and this may help in the differentiation, but in the end it may not be possible with these three simple tests to be absolutely sure what is going on and further help will then be needed.

Glossopharyngeal and vagus nerves (IX, X)

Together these two nerves supply sensation to the skin of the posterior wall of the ear canal and the adjacent portion of the pinna, and sensation to the mucosa of the soft palate, palatal arches, and pharynx. They also innervate the muscles of the palatal arches, the muscles that elevate the palate and the muscles of the pharynx although the contribution from each nerve is still a matter for discussion. The vagus is the prime mover of the vocal cords whilst the glossopharyngeal supplies taste from the posterior third of the tongue. The vagus has a further wide distribution, that need not bother us here. The motor function of the two nerves are the easiest to assess. Lesions of the vagus or glossopharyngeal nuclei in the brainstem or of the nerves themselves close to the base of the skull cause a paralysis of the palate and pharynx. When the patient is asked to say 'ah' the palate elevates and deviates to the normal side. Sensation is also lost in this region and can be assessed by light touch with a cotton bud. The combination of poor movement and sensation may cause major difficulties in swallowing food and liquids, especially, may be regurgitated into the post-nasal space. So far it is not possible to differentiate between disorders of IX and X but a lesion of X will, in addition, cause a weak or hoarse voice and an examination of the larynx using a headlight and mirror, or a flexible fibreoptic telescope will reveal a cord palsy or weakness on speaking, thereby confirming the lesion. Anyone who has been hoarse for, say, six weeks or more must have examination of the larynx to rule out a laryngeal tumour, even if other causes are suspected.

The accessory (XI)

The accessory supplies the sternomastoid and trapezius muscles and is tested, first, by asking the patient to push his forehead forward against the palm of his or your hand whilst you feel for the contraction in the sternomastoid muscles in the root of the neck and, second, by asking them to shrug their shoulders. A unilateral loss or weakness is usually easily recognised (Figure 4.24).

The hypoglossal (XII)

The hypoglossal is the motor nerve to the tongue and is tested by examining the mobility of the tongue. Ask the patient to open their mouth and poke the tongue straight out. It will deviate to the same side as the lesion in the nerve. They will be unable to move the tongue to the unaffected side, or at least the mobility will be much reduced. In a lesion of the nerve itself (a

Figure 4.24: Testing for contraction of the sternomastoid. By asking the patient to push against the examiner's hand the sternomastoids are made to contract and can be seen and should also be felt to detect assymetry in their tension.

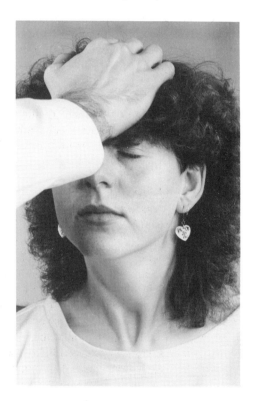

lower motor neurone lesion) there may, in addition, be wasting of the tongue and fasciculation visible on the surface after the nerve has been non-functioning for some time. The tongue lies unhappily in the floor of the mouth with one side shrunken, frequently wrinkled and often gently twitching.

THE PERIPHERAL NERVOUS SYSTEM

Within the context of the examination for dizziness, testing peripheral sensation is more rewarding than a detailed assessment of power, tone and the reflexes. Edwards (1973) suggests that the best single test is that of vibration perception using a low frequency 128 Hz tuning fork. Set the tuning fork vibrating and first of all apply the base to the top end of the sternum so that the patient understands the sensation we are testing. In the normal, the sensation should be equal when the tuning fork is placed first on the big toe and then on the thumb. With old age, the ability to perceive vibration may decline, first in the feet, then at the ankle and calf but this loss should not reach the knee.

This form of testing is, of course, subjective and all sorts of misunderstanding can arise. However, by sometimes having the tuning fork vibrating and sometimes not, it is usually possible to overcome these problems of communication and reach a valid result.

THE CARDIOVASCULAR SYSTEM

Do take the blood pressure and feel the pulse. It is so easy to do and can provide many answers. If there is any suggestion of a postural element, take the blood pressure with the patient lying on a couch and then again very shortly after he has stood up. Listen to the heart especially carefully if the history is suggestive of transient cerebral ischaemia as valvular disease may well be a cause, as can atheroma in the carotids, sometimes detectable by an audible bruit with the stethoscope placed lightly on the front of the sternomastoid on each side. Other less common conditions such as the subclavian steal syndrome (Chapter 14) can be suggested by the history and the diagnosis strengthened by finding different blood pressures in each arm and perhaps a weaker pulse on the affected side. The list can go on but naturally your examination is directed by the history and more specific findings will therefore be described in the relevant sections later in the book.

EXAMINATION OF THE EAR

Frequently vertigo is caused by disease in the ear. Sometimes the culprit can be seen simply by looking with an auriscope. To examine the adult ear, first, look at the external ear then turn it forward to see if there are scars over the mastoid prominence indicating previous operations. To look into the ear canal in the adult you need to straighten out the curve of the cartilaginous ear canal and to do this the pinna is gently pulled backwards and upwards. With a suitable sized speculum on the auriscope you should guide the tip into the ear canal and then look through the lens to follow the ear canal. The eardrum is placed a little anteriorly so that the auriscope has to be angled forwards. Clinical notes sometimes contain the record — 'Eardrum dull, red and featureless'. It may be dull and red but it is never featureless, and the author of the observation has probably been looking at the posterior canal wall. Usually you cannot see all of the eardrum at the same time so it is probably best to use a landmark to guide you. The one landmark that seems constant in spite of disease, is the lateral process of the malleus (Figure 4.25). Find this first then look in different directions to examine all of the eardrum and especially the region above the malleus handle — the attic, for this is frequently the site of disease that is notorious for causing serious complications, including vertigo.

Some auriscopes have little pneumatic puffers attached to them and you should puff air into the ear canal via the speculum to see if the eardrum moves — which is the normal response.

When you have finished looking remove the auriscope and test for the presence of a fistula into the inner ear. Ask the patient to look straight ahead and tell them that you are going to press on the ear. Then, with a finger press on the tragus so that it occludes the canal, and then press a little harder to raise the pressure in the ear canal. Practice on yourself to get the idea of how hard to push without causing pain. A positive fistula sign occurs when the eyes deviate away from the side under test. The patient may also feel vertiginous. Release the pressure and the eyes return usually with a few beats of nystagmus. A positive fistula sign nearly always indicates underlying disease that requires further investigation and may well need treatment.

When you have finished on one side examine the other, even if you have found obvious pathology.

In babies and infants the ear canal has a different curvature and to see the eardrum the external ear has to be gently pulled down and back. The eardrum is full size at birth, as is the middle ear and its contents, but the angle of the ear canal can make it difficult to see.

Figure 4.25: The right tympanic membrane. This photograph has been taken using a wide angle endoscope and it is rarely possible to see all the drum like this with an auriscope. The malleus handle runs from the centre of the drum upwards and apparently fowards to the prominent lateral process. Above this is the pars flaccida and below the pars tensa. Although the annulus of the drum can be seen, black and white photography does not do justice to the subject.

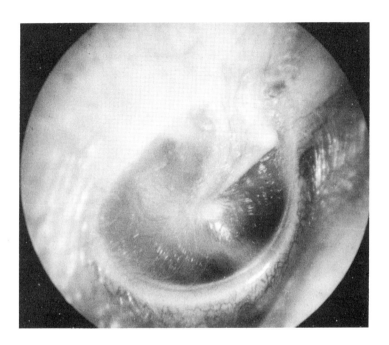

THE INVESTIGATIONS

During the course of your history and examination you may uncover something that needs referral or specialist attention. Some simple investigations nevertheless provide a baseline from which many conditions can be excluded or confirmed. A full blood count (FBC), microscopy of the film and an erythrocyte sedimentation rate (ESR) is very valuable. At the same time blood should also be taken for a blood sugar estimate and serology test for syphilis. The best single test for syphilis is probably the Fluorescent Treponemal Antibody absorption test (FTA-Abs) and this should always be requested.

The results of the FBC and film may prompt further investigations such as estimation of the iron, folate and B_{12}, or blood alcohol levels but it would seem more sensible to investigate abnormalities sequentially rather than to send off a bucket of blood for every test known to man, and hope you turn up something abnormal.

SUMMARY

Having read the chapter on the history and examination you probably feel that the whole thing is quite unmanageable in a busy clinic or surgery. However, with organisation of your examination routine, so that unnecessary or repetitive manoeuvres are avoided, the procedure can be quite quick, especially when you develop your own technique and modify the examination in the light of the history. A scheme for organising the examination that has the patient sitting, standing then lying on a couch seems to minimise the time for the examination and is presented in Table 4.8.

Table 4.8: Scheme for assessment of the dizzy patient

1. History		
2. Examination	Patient sitting	Check ears
		Test hearing
		Check cranial nerves
		Look for spontaneous nystagmus
		Use ophthalmoscope
		Check co-ordination
		Take B.P. and pulse
	Patient standing	Romberg's test
		Gait
		Walk to couch
	Patient on couch	Positional tests first
		Test vibration sense
		Listen to heart and chest
		Check pulse
		Lying/Standing B.P.
		Cool calorics
3. Investigation		Take bloods
	may decide on	CXR, ECG, Audiograms
		Bithermal calorics

It has been said that if you do not have any idea of the diagnosis or at least where the trouble lies, by the time you have finished taking the history then, however diligent your examination, you are unlikely to make further progress. This does seem to hold true and taking a good history will usually save time and money being spent on unnecessary investigation.

5

The Ear and its Diseases

In the majority of patients with vertigo and in many with unsteadiness the ear will be found to be at the root of the problem. In the chapters that follow the major ear conditions that result in 'dizziness' will be described. Of course, there are many other conditions that occasionally cause problems and some of these are brought together to form a miscellaneous collection at the end of this section.

Table 5.1 indicates the range of conditions covered. This chapter takes you gently through the anatomy of the ear and deals with middle ear disease.

Subsequent chapters describe the rest of the range of conditions whilst Chapter 18 contains a section on the drug management of dizziness and gives a protocol for vestibular exercises that have been found to be useful in rehabilitation.

A SIMPLE ANATOMY OF THE EAR

The ear is conveniently described in three portions being outer, middle and inner. The inner ear has already been mentioned in Chapter 1, and the outer ear comprising, the auricle and ear canal, is not often relevant to the discussion of vertigo so that we can concentrate on the middle ear.

The middle ear can be thought of as a room with four walls, a ceiling and a floor. If you imagine yourself standing in this room representing the right ear, and facing forwards then the relationship of various structures becomes easy (Figure 5.1). To your right hand is the eardrum, and through that the external ear canal. In front of you is a bony wall with the opening of the

Table 5.1: Ear conditions resulting in vertigo

Middle ear disease:	Acute suppurative otitis media
	Chronic suppurative otitis media
	serous labyrinthitis
	suppurative labyrinthitis
	Cholesteatoma
	... Chapter 5
Trauma to the inner ear:	Surgical
	Direct trauma to the head
	Pressure-induced damage
	... Chapter 6
Ménière's disease and syndrome	... Chapter 7
Benign paroxysmal positional vertigo	... Chapter 8
Vestibular neuronitis and the Ramsay-Hunt Syndrome	... Chapter 9
Syphilis	... Chapter 10
Miscellaneous ear conditions:	Wax
	Otosclerosis
	Paget's disease
	Drugs damaging the labyrinth
	... Chapter 11

Figure 5.1: Structures lying next to the right middle ear.

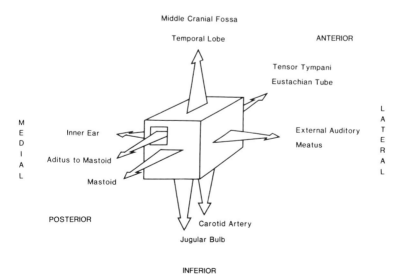

87

Eustachian tube half way up leading forwards into the naso-pharynx. Through the wall on your left hand is the inner ear, with the bony labyrinth being represented by two swellings on your side of this wall. The front one is the bone over the basal turn of the cochlea — the promontory, and the back one the dome of the lateral semicircular canal is on the top back corner of this left hand wall. Also on this wall and just behind the promontory are two windows into the labyrinth. The oval window is sealed by the bony footplate of the stapes and lies above the round window which is closed by a thin membrane only four or five cell layers thick, but protected by a bony over-hang. The back wall of the middle ear separates you from the mastoid air cells but there is on the top inner corner an opening called the aditus to the mastoid.

Beneath your feet is the jugular vein as it arches up to form the jugular bulb and ahead of this and in the front wall of the middle ear is the carotid artery as it turns forward in the skull to run alongside the Eustachian tube.

Over your head is an incomplete false ceiling consisting of several folds of mucosa running from the eardrum to the inner bony wall. The space above this is the attic region, actually named this, and surrounded by bone. Through its thin bony roof is the dura of the middle cranial fossa and the temporal lobe of the brain.

The middle ear space contains the three ossicles — malleus, incus and stapes — that connect the eardrum to the inner ear and convert air-borne sound into pressure waves within the cochlear fluids. These are subsequently detected by the sensory cells of the organ of Corti, and transmitted by the acoustic nerve to the brainstem (Figure 5.2).

The handle of the malleus lies within the eardrum with its prominent lateral process forming a useful landmark when the ear is examined with an auriscope. The head of the malleus which arises from the handle by way of a narrow neck, is above you in the attic region draped by the various membranes and supporting ligaments. There is a synovial joint on the back surface of the malleus to connect with the head of the incus. This is also suspended in the attic by membranes and ligaments. From the head of the incus one long process passes down and articulates with the head of the stapes. This is connected via an arch of bone to the footplate, sitting in the oval window and connected by a thin membrane to the bony edges of the window. A short process projects backwards from the head of the incus to just enter the aditus to the mastoid air cell system.

The mastoid bone contains a honeycomb of interconnected air-filled spaces that varies in size from a small cavity surrounded by dense bone in some people to an extensive space surrounded by a thin shell in others. The relationships of important structures to the right mastoid are shown in Figure 5.3.

For completeness the course of the facial nerve through the middle ear space will be described. It makes its appearance near the front of the medial wall of the middle ear, just above the promontory. This is the site of the geniculate ganglion and it is marked on the bony wall by a small curved bony out-growth, the processus cochleariformis (nothing to do with the cochlea — but

Figure 5.2: Two views of the right middle ear.
m = malleus, i = incus, et = Eustachian tube, j = jugular bulb, c = carotid artery, s = stapes, VII = VIIn nerve, LC = lateral semicircular canal.
(a) Looking outwards from the middle ear shows the eardrum with the malleus handle embedded in it and the heads of the malleus and incus located in the attic. The roof of the middle ear is very thin and in some ears, especially those of children, is deficient. The Eustachian tube runs forwards from the middle ear.

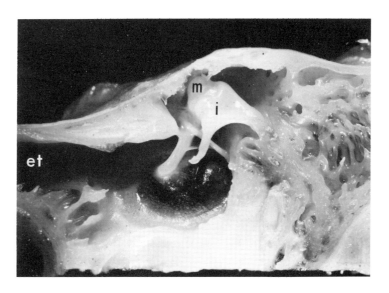

(b) Looking inwards to show the jugular bulb and carotid artery in the floor of the middle ear. The stapes is seen with the short stapedius tendon and just above this and curving down is the facial nerve. Above and slightly behind the facial nerve is the smooth dome of the lateral semicircular canal. Above this again is the opening into the mastoid with its honeycomb-like collection of air cells.

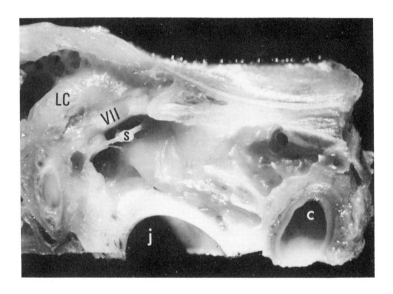

so-named because it is spoon-shaped). The facial nerve lies in a prominent yet thin-walled bony tunnel that runs back just above the oval window and below the dome of the lateral semicircular canal. It then turns downwards into the thicker bone between the mastoid and middle ear to leave the base of the skull through the stylo-mastoid foramen. In its descent it gives off a small branch to supply the stapedius muscle and a bigger branch — the chorda tympani — which carries taste fibres from the anterior two-third of the tongue. To get to the tongue the nerve passes obliquely forwards and upwards and has to cross the middle ear which it does within the layers of the eardrum, running behind the neck of the malleus.

The stapedius muscle runs from the back wall of the middle ear to the head of the stapes and its contraction stiffens the stapes and reduces its mobility although its function in life is still speculative. There is another muscle in the middle ear. This is

Figure 5.3: Relationships of right mastoid cavity.

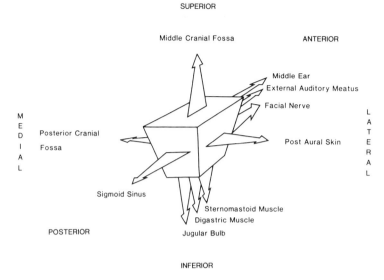

the tensor tympani and it runs from a canal in the roof of the Eustachian tube back to the processus cochleariformis where its tendon, held down by a ligament running across this structure, turns through 90 degrees to reach the back of the neck of the malleus. It, like the stapedius, acts to stiffen up the ossicular chain but again without any proven use.

MIDDLE EAR DISEASE

(Colour plates showing normal and diseased eardrums appear at the end of the chapter)

The normal middle ear and mastoid is an air-filled bony box connected to the nasopharynx by the Eustachian tube. It has one flexible wall, the eardrum. Oxygen is resorbed by the mucosa lining these cavities so that the air pressure slowly falls with time. This is corrected every few minutes by swallowing, which opens the Eustachian tube by the pull of the palatal and pharyngeal muscles and allows a small amount of air to pass into the middle ear. The volumes involved are very small with a number of studies finding that about 1 ml of air enters the

91

middle ear via the Eustachian tube each day (see Sade 1979). With Eustachian tube dysfunction, whatever its cause, ventilation of the middle ear becomes inadequate and a number of conditions may arise.

We are all probably familiar with the temporary failure that occurs following a viral upper respiratory tract infection. There is congestion and over-production of the normal secretions from the respiratory mucosa lining the Eustachian tube and that portion of the middle ear mucose close to its opening. These secretions may fill up the middle ear and the eardrum becomes retracted as the middle ear pressure falls. The result is muffled hearing, a feeling of pressure or discomfort in the ear and sometimes clicking or gurgling noises as the fluid moves around. This condition is called a secretory otitis media, it is very common and usually resolves quite quickly as the Eustachian tube recovers.

When the function of the Eustachian tube is impaired for longer periods, the condition becomes established. There is a change in the consistency of the fluid in the middle ear — it becomes thicker and viscid — and alterations to the mucosa of the middle ear which become more 'respiratory' in nature. This longstanding secretory otitis media rejoices under a plethora of names with 'middle ear effusion' and 'otitis media with effusion' currently being fashionable, although the term 'glue ear' has stuck in the literature. There are some specific causes of glue ear, with cleft palate and cystic fibrosis usually being associated with the condition, and tumours in the post-nasal space sometimes causing trouble in one ear. These diseases are uncommon, whilst the incidence of glue ear in childhood is high and presumably the underlying cause of the Eustachian tube dysfunction is multifactorial with enlarged adenoids, recurrent infection, allergy and an immature shape and function of the tube all playing a so far undefinable part.

In childhood the condition presents with recurrent earache, hearing loss that is initially fluctuating but then becomes established, possibly a slowness in acquiring, or a deterioration of speech and perhaps inattention or naughtiness at school. The eardrum is retracted, dull, sometimes bluish and there are usually prominent radial blood vessels visible. As the child grows the condition tends to resolve as the various underlying conditions regress and the Eustachian tube improves.

However, several complications can arise. The fluid that is

present can become infected, usually by *Haemophilus influenzae* or *Streptococcus pneumoniae* ascending the Eustachian tube, and result in an acute suppurative otitis media. This can occur both in the glue ear child and in anyone with an acute secretory otitis media. There is increasing pain, a worsening of the hearing and, as the eardrum starts to bulge under the pressure of the inflammatory exudate and pus, a little watery or even blood-stained discharge from the ear may be noticed. Then the eardrum bursts, the pain is relieved and a sticky mucopus runs out of the ear canal. The middle ear is now ventilated again, the condition settles and the eardrum usually heals. Children may therefore have recurrent bouts of a purulent discharge from the middle ear as the cycle repeats itself — the underlying cause of the Eustachian tube dysfunction still being present.

Occasionally the perforation persists and the ear can either remain dry or become permanently or intermittently wet if the middle ear mucosa has undergone change to a respiratory type epithelium — rather like the condition in a chronic bronchitic. The perforation in all these cases is in the central portion of the eardrum and this condition is a so-called 'safe-type' of chronic suppurative otitis media, for although it may be unpleasant with an intermittent purulent discharge and deafness, serious complications are few and far between.

However, another form of chronic ear disease can develop from persisting Eustachian tube dysfunction. With the continued lowered middle ear pressure the drum can become retracted and stuck down onto the medial wall of the middle ear. Adhesions can also form between the walls of the middle ear cavity and the mucosal folds and ossicles contained within its spaces, rather like the adhesions that occur following intra-abdominal surgery or infection. Both adhesions and retractions result in parts of the middle ear being further isolated from the Eustachian tube so that the drum covering these parts of the middle ear continue to be drawn in and retraction pockets develop. This process is insidious and once started seems to carry on under its own steam so that the original conditions that caused the glue ear have often resolved and fluid is no longer apparent in the middle ear. Sometimes the gross features of glue ear are never present, just a slowly developing retraction with an occasional ear infection during childhood. The posterior superior portion of the tense part of the drum, and the superior or attic regions of the drum are usually involved in the develop-

93

ment of these retraction pockets.

The normal eardrum is covered by a thin layer of skin, and this layer, like skin anywhere, continues to grow and shed sheets of desquamated keratin. In the eardrum, however, there is radial migration of the surface layers to the edge of the eardrum where, along with the skin of the ear canal, migration to the external opening of the ear canal occurs. The result is the white flaky material — rather like dandruff — that you find on the tip of your finger when you scratch your ear; a habit not to be encouraged.

Retraction pockets can prevent the efficient migration of the desquamated skin which therefore builds up within the pocket, eventually to form a solid plug of white keratin. The skin surrounding this is continuing to grow and therefore has to expand to accommodate the ever-increasing mass of debris. This sac of skin filled with keratin is called a cholesteatoma and it grows into the surrounding cavities and takes up the shape of the space in which it finds itself. Eventually something happens to change the properties of the cholesteatoma and it starts actively to erode the nearby bone. There are other theories about the formation of the cholesteatoma with direct growth of the skin at the margins of the eardrum into the middle ear spaces being one.

Whatever the precise cause of the disease, cholesteatoma can cause problems because of the close proximity of important structures to the middle ear. It can erode through the roof of the middle ear and mastoid to reach the middle cranial fossa, through the medial wall of the mastoid to involve the posterior fossa, into the facial nerve, and importantly for this book, through the bony labyrinth and into the inner ear. Deafness can also arise because the ossicles are eroded or fixed by the mass of keratin. The cholesteatoma can itself become infected, frequently with a mixture of anaerobes and Gram-negative bacteria to produce a foul-smelling discharge. This final complication is again a chronic suppurative otitis media but now it is unsafe.

Figure 5.4 is a flow chart of the possible routes to both safe and unsafe ear disease.

Dizziness can make an appearance at various stages in the development of chronic middle ear disease.

Figure 5.4: Flow chart of possible routes from a normal ear with Eustachian tube dysfunction to various types of ear disease.

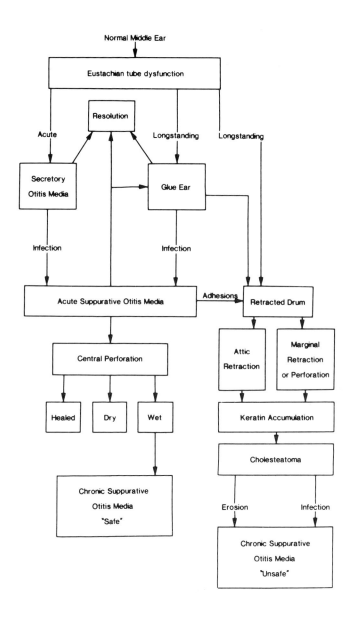

GLUE EAR

When the middle ear is full of glue and the eardrum is retracted, children sometimes become and feel unsteady and fall about. They rarely have vertiginous symptoms and are usually able to distinguish the symptoms of unsteadiness from those of vertigo by analogy to the roundabouts and the sensation that comes on after whirling themselves around. Presumably the unsteadiness occurs because the middle ear pressure changes are transmitted to the inner ear via the oval and round windows.

There are no medications that have been properly shown to influence the natural history of glue ear, nor to bring short-term improvement. Treatment if needed is surgical. Incision of the eardrum (myringotomy) and aspiration of the glue is the initial step. Most surgeons insert a ventilation tube (grommet) into the eardrum to bypass the malfunctioning Eustachian tube, and many will remove the adenoids at the same operation. The unsteadiness is nearly always resolved by the insertion of the grommet.

ACUTE SUPPURATIVE OTITIS MEDIA

All sorts of dizziness can arise during the course of an acute otitis media. During the preceding viral infection, with fever and a tachycardia, light-headedness can occur on rapid changes of position. When the middle ear is full of fluid whether it be infected or not, unsteadiness can arise on top of the light-headedness. Occasionally vertigo can develop when there is pus in the middle ear. Presumably the local hyperaemia and irritation can affect the perilymph and endolymph and the term serous labyrinthitis is applied to this condition. It usually occurs in one ear and the patient, in addition to the bulging red eardrum, has a sensorineural hearing loss that can be impossible to detect without audiometric help as there is already a conductive loss. A spontaneous vestibular type horizontal nystagmus is usually present. In the early stages, the irritation of the labyrinth drives the eyes away from the affected ear so that the fast phase of the nystagmus is towards this side, rather like the warm caloric test. If the vestibular labyrinth subsequently dies the nystagmus will reverse direction so that the eyes are pushed towards the affected ear by the unopposed activity of the healthy ear. This is like the nystagmus seen during a cool caloric test with the fast phase away from the diseased ear. The appearance of vertigo and nystagmus during this sort of condition can raise the possibility of an acute suppurative labyrinthitis. The distinction is, however, of little importance since the management is the same whether the problem is serous or suppurative and indeed labels can only be applied in retrospect when investigations show either a dead ear and no vestibular function (suppurative) or some hearing and a caloric response (serous).

Treatment comprises bed rest, analgesics, antibiotics and vestibular sedatives. If the eardrum has not perforated spontaneously a myringotomy is needed to drain the pus which should be cultured and the antibiotics adjusted according to the sensitivity report.

CHRONIC SUPPURATIVE OTITIS MEDIA

Safe type

In those ears with a wet central perforation and a thickened red granular mucosa lining the middle ear space, the development of an infection on top of the mucous discharge can often result in unsteadiness and sometimes bouts of vertigo, especially on head movement. Presumably there is a serous labyrinthitis at work and this will continue to irritate the inner ear until the infection settles. The patient's history of a longstanding mucoid discharge, allied with seeing a central perforation and being positive that there is no serious ear disease present, will allow you to treat this with antibiotic ear drops, perhaps oral antibiotics, if there is an obvious local cellulitis, and some vestibular sedatives to help the patient over the acute phase. If you are unhappy about the condition of the eardrum, especially the attic regions the patient should be referred to an ear, nose and throat clinic.

If the attacks of vertigo recur with each episode of suppuration then it is sometimes possible to explore the mastoid and middle ear spaces, to remove the diseased mucosa and graft the hole in the eardrum. This procedure is often successful in preventing the recurrent discharge and stopping the vertigo but like all major ear surgery it is not without its risks of a sensorineural deafness, a facial palsy, a worsened vertigo, tinnitus and

97

even persistent discharge if the graft fails. These and the risks of the anaesthetic may outweigh the possible benefits, especially in the elderly.

Unsafe type

Bouts of short-lived vertigo, accompanied by unsteadiness, that develop during chronic middle ear disease, should always raise the possibility of an erosive cholesteatoma in your mind. There need not have been any other ear symptoms, the patient not noticing a minimal conductive loss or neglecting an occasional bout of discomfort in the ear. A slowly growing cholesteatoma, that does not get infected can easily erode the lateral semi-circular canal so that a labyrinthine fistula develops without other symptoms. Usually, however, the patient has had foul discharge from the ear, some hearing loss and perhaps a dull ache in the ear or on the side of the head because of the osteitis.

On examination, the lower portion of the drum may be quite normal with there being just a small crust of wax over the attic region. This attic wax must be removed to see what is going on underneath and however suggestive the symptoms are of another disease the patient should be seen by an ENT surgeon who, using suction and an operating microscope, can carefully examine the suspicious areas. The fistula test described in Chapter 4 may be positive and there is frequently some conductive hearing loss. The cholesteatoma may on the other hand be quite obvious, and again the patient needs referral since the treatment of this condition is nearly always surgical, with some form of mastoidectomy being needed in most cases. It is usually possible to preserve cochlear and labyrinthine function at mastoidectomy in spite of a fistula, although the growth of cholesteatoma into the inner ear may make conservation difficult. A surgical dilemma arises if the ear with a cholesteatoma causing vertigo is the only ear with any useful hearing.

An infected cholesteatoma and a labyrinthine fistula can cause a suppurative labyrinthitis. Untreated, the chances of preservation of hearing are slight and so it seems sensible to operate under antibiotic cover to remove the nidus of infection in the hope of preserving some hearing at least.

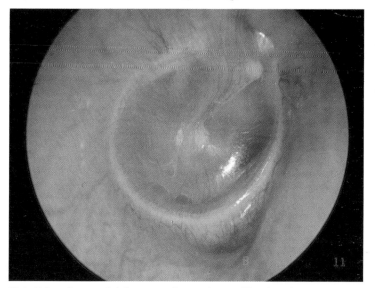

Plate 5.1a: A normal right tympanic membrane. The drum is thin and translucent. The malleus handle lies within the drum and runs from the centre to the 'one o'clock' position. At its upper end is the prominent, white lateral process, which is a reliable landmark. Behind the malleus handle can just be seen the lower end of the long process of the incus.

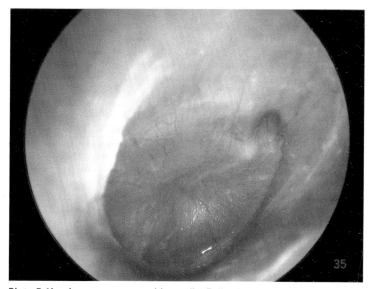

Plate 5.1b: Acute secretory otitis media. Following an upper respiratory tract infection the drum has become slightly retracted, has lost its transparency and has acquired a glistening appearance.

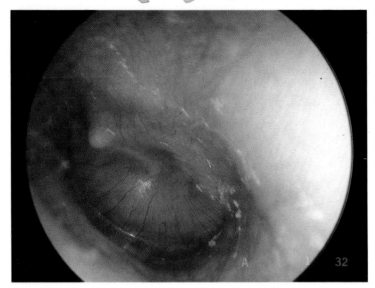

Plate 5.2a: Chronic secretory otitis media — glue ear. The drum is dull, retracted and almost bluish in colour. Radial blood vessels are clearly visible.

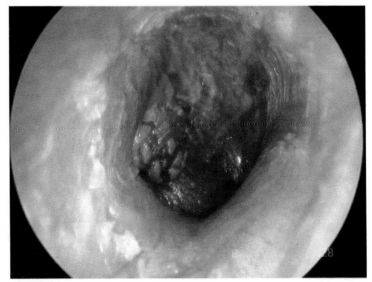

Plate 5.2b: Acute suppurative otitis media. Here the fluid in the middle ear has become infected and pus has formed so that the posterior part of the drum is bulging and is about ready to perforate spontaneously.

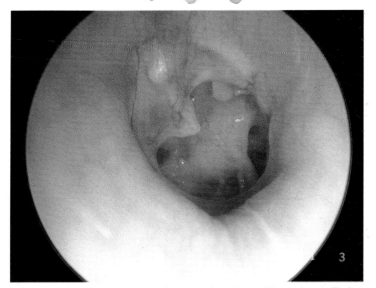

Plate 5.3a: A large, but dry, perforation of the drum. The patient is likely to have a hearing loss, could have recurrent discharge and tinnitus, but might well be symptom free. This is a 'safe', central type perforation.

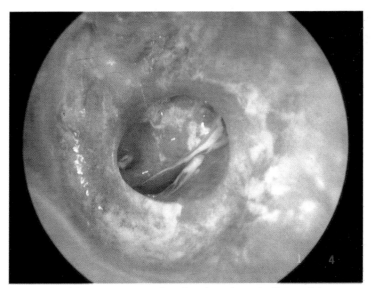

Plate 5.3b: A large, wet, central perforation where the lining of the middle ear has undergone a change into a thickened, moist respiratory type mucosa that constantly discharges and is sometimes infected.

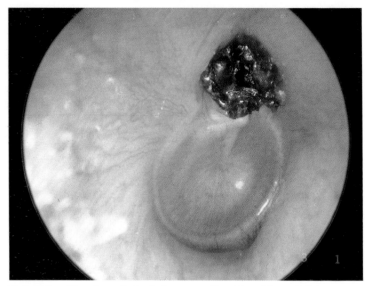

Plate 5.4a: Unsafe — cholesteatoma ear. Over the attic part of the ear drum is a crust which covers a cholesteatoma. The patient may be asymptomatic if the disease is limited, but can develop deafness, vertigo, a facial palsy or even an intracranial complication as extension and bone erosion takes place.

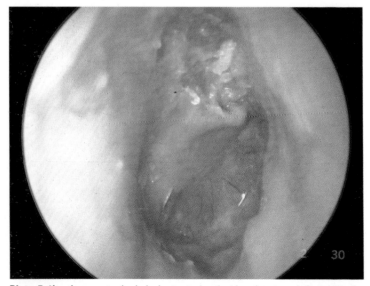

Plate 5.4b: A more typical cholesteatoma that has become infected and is producing a foul smelling discharge. The white debris above the lateral process of the malleus is the desquamated skin that forms the core of the cholesteatoma.

6

Trauma to the Inner Ear

The majority of cases of trauma to the inner ear are caused by surgeons operating on the middle ear, or by direct injuries to the head. Occasionally pressure changes cause trouble and this chapter will deal with these major groups in order.

SURGICAL TRAUMA

During surgery to the middle ear and mastoid there is always the risk of coming across an asymptomatic fistula into the inner ear. This is frequently the result of longstanding cholesteatoma but sometimes occurs in 'safe' middle ear disease with only infected granulations. Failure to recognise this fistula and the subsequent suction on the perilymph nearly always results in severe post-operative vertigo with a typical vestibular-type horizontal nystagmus of variable degree which slowly fades over a number of days or perhaps weeks. When the labyrinth is dead the fast phase of the nystagmus is away from the operated ear. The vertigo rarely lasts without break for more than a day or two, but is easily brought on by head movements during the next few days, and unsteadiness persists until compensation is complete. Usually the cochlear portion of the labyrinth is affected as well, with a sensorineural hearing loss directing the Weber test to the unoperated ear. This loss can be complete or partial and does not improve. It appears to be the suction on the perilymph that does the damage, rather than the uncomplicated opening of the inner ear. There is continuing argument as to whether cholesteatoma should be removed from a fistula, which is then closed with fascia, albeit with the risk of a dead ear, or left as a small patch after the surrounding mass of keratin has been removed. The conservative approach is justified if there is no useful hearing in the other ear, but many surgeons report preservation of hearing if the cholesteatoma is removed very carefully without suction on the perilymph. An individual's practice seems to be the outcome of their earlier teaching, their technical skills and experience so that no firm guidelines can really be given here.

During the operation of stapedectomy (or stapedotomy) for otosclerosis, the footplate of the stapes is removed completely (-ectomy) or a small hole made in it (-otomy), so that direct communication is made with the perilymph. This opening is then filled up with some form of prosthetic device that is attached to the long process of the incus. This allows vibration to be transmitted directly to the perilymph, thereby sidestepping the bony overgrowth of the stapes footplate that causes the conductive deafness of otosclerosis (Figure 6.1 and Chapter 11). Following this procedure, even in the hands of the best surgeon and when the operation has gone smoothly, transitory vertigo, accompanied by nystagmus, is common although major sensorineural hearing loss is fortunately less often seen.

During other procedures on the middle ear the ossicular chain can be knocked during manipulation or the vibration of the drill transmitted to the inner ear more than it can tolerate. The vertigo that results from this form of trauma is fortunately short-lived, and the nystagmus suggestive of an irritative lesion with the fast phase towards the operated ear. Fortunately, the vertigo and unsteadiness settle rapidly, especially in the younger patient.

The persistence or development of an intermittent post-operative vertigo especially when associated with lying flat, coughing, or straining to rid oneself of the constipation that follows the use of narcotic analgesics, should raise the suggestion of a labyrinthine fistula, especially if associated with a sensorineural hearing loss. This may be expected from the operative findings or comes as a surprise to both surgeon and patient. The management can be a problem. In the first place, fistulae will sometimes heal themselves, and so a period of bed rest with vestibular sedatives and antibiotics to guard against a suppurative labyrinthitis, is indicated. Many will settle after a few days, but some will not and may prompt the surgeon to re-explore the ear especially if the hearing is deteriorating. If a

Figure 6.1: Diagram representing the end result of a stapedotomy with a prosthetic replacement of the stapes superstructure. A hole is made in the footplate and there is the possibility of direct damage to the underlying labyrinth during the procedure, or of a subsequent leak of perilymph.

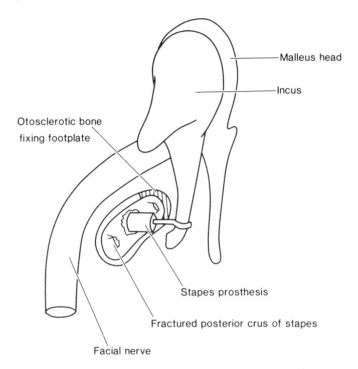

Malleus head

Incus

Otosclerotic bone fixing footplate

Stapes prosthesis

Fractured posterior crus of stapes

Facial nerve

fistula is found it can be sealed with fascia or a plug of fat, but there is always the risk of converting a hearing ear into a dead ear, however careful the exploration. This is especially so following a stapedectomy as manipulation around the footplate is notorious for causing further, perhaps complete, deafness. A further dilemma arises if the ear with the fistula is the only hearing ear when the balance is between whether to leave the fistula and risk a dead ear, or operate and risk the same.

Some time after mastoid and middle ear surgery vertigo can arise for a number of reasons other than those described above. Persisting disease in a mastoid cavity with recurrent cholesteatoma or infected granulations can cause vertigo either because of a slow erosion into the labyrinth or because a serous labyrinthitis develops. Here the mastoid cavity is wet, there may be

101

obvious disease and a fistula test might be positive. In either case, a surgical revision of the mastoid is needed if only to exclude a fistula and remove infected granulations. The granulations should always be sent for histology as carcinoma is sometimes found in a longstanding wet mastoid cavity and needs further treatment which is frequently and unfortunately only palliative. Recurrent cholesteatoma should be treated as if it were fresh disease and the management of a fistula rests on the principles laid out before, and upon the skill of the surgeon.

Even in dry mastoid cavities, especially in those where the external ear canal has been extensively enlarged, vertigo can arise when cold winds or hot or cold water unexpectedly enters the cavity. Here there is a direct caloric effect, at least on the lateral semicircular canal which is unprotected by the mass of surrounding mastoid bone. This can cause problems if the individual is riding his bicycle in heavy traffic or is misguidedly swimming in deep water as orientation is upset and disasters have sometimes occurred. The diagnosis is usually obvious and the cure is avoidance with ear plugs, ear muffs, scarves or common sense.

Vertigo and unsteadiness can also arise many years after surgery which resulted in a dead ear with loss of vestibular function. This is rather like the unsteadiness that sometimes develops twenty or so years after a bout of vestibular neuronitis (Chapter 9) when the ageing vestibular system is unable to cope with the stress of sudden movement, being deprived of useful information from the dead labyrinth. Provided other causes of vertigo are excluded and the mastoid cavity is clean and dry, a course of vestibular exercises are often useful. The absence of vestibular function must be made positively by the lack of response on a cool then cold caloric test if the eardrum is intact. If there is a mastoid cavity then a modification of the test, using cold air rather than water, should also show a lack of response.

Finally, intermittent bouts of vertigo, unrelated to but made worse by head movement and associated with a feeling of fullness or pressure in the ear, can rarely arise twenty or more years following a mastoidectomy or other surgical procedure which resulted in a severe sensorineural hearing loss but no permanent vestibular damage. It is thought that a series of changes occur in the labyrinth not unlike those that arise in Ménière's disease (Chapter 7). There is dilation of the membranous labyrinth with presumably over-accumulation of endolymph, resulting in minute pressure changes that causes bouts of vertigo. The condition is dignified by the title 'delayed endolymphatic hydrops' and since there is no useful hearing then the treatment that works is surgical destruction of the labyrinth — a labyrinthectomy. Vertigo persisting after a labyrinthectomy, for whatever reason it was performed, suggests either that the operation was inadequate with residual intact nerve endings, that the other ear was also involved, or that the diagnosis was wrong.

DIRECT TRAUMA TO THE HEAD

Direct trauma to the head and neck can result in a wide variety of problems including vertigo (Table 6.1). In this section we will deal with fractures of the temporal bone and concussion to the central vestibular pathways. Injuries causing benign paroxysmal positional vertigo are dealt with in Chapter 8, whiplash injuries to the neck in Chapter 13 and ruptures of the labyrinthine membranes in the next section of this chapter.

Fractures of the temporal bone

Injuries severe enough to cause fractures which pass through the temporal bone are often associated with other major trauma so that the deafness and vertigo that result are of minor consequence in the early acute phase, but may form a serious and often neglected problem in the recovery stage. The early management of major head injury is outside the scope of this book but sometimes direct blows to the side of the head will cause temporal bone damage with few other injuries. The symptoms and signs that result from this lesser trauma are also

Table 6.1: Causes of vertigo following trauma to the head

Fractures of the temporal bone	... Chapter 6
Concussion to brainstem and cerebellum	... Chapter 6
Whiplash injuries to the neck	... Chapter 12
Benign paroxysmal positional vertigo	... Chpater 8
Rupture of labyrinthine membranes and barotrauma	... Chapter 6

found in the more major injuries and will be helpful in the initial assessment.

Temporal bone fractures are classed as longitudinal, transverse or mixed. The terms longitudinal and transverse relate to the long axis of the petrous portion of the temporal bone, which contains the middle and inner ears, and is more or less pyramid shaped with the pointed end forwards. Running along the long axis of this pyramid are a number of cavities with the mastoid at the back, the outer and middle ear spaces centrally and the Eustachian tube and carotid canal at the front. Longitudinal fractures extend, in general, from the flat squamous portion of the temporal bone through the posterior superior portion of the external ear canal, across the roof of the middle ear and then along the line of the Eustachian tube and carotid canal to end in the middle cranial fossa near the foramen spinosum through which passes the middle meningeal artery (Figure 6.2).

Transverse fractures run across the long axis of the bone and can take a variety of pathways from the foramen magnum to the middle cranial fossa via the numerous foramina that exist in the temporal bone, so that separate fragments of bone are sometimes produced. A typical fracture would be from the foramen magnum to the jugular foramen and hypoglossal (XII) nerve canal, through the internal auditory meatus to end in the middle cranial fossa in the region of the foramen lacerum, through which passes the internal carotid artery. En route it breaks open the bony labyrinth (Figure 6.3).

Mixed fractures resulting from severe crushing head injuries are a combination of the above two with a mixture of the signs and symptoms and will not be discussed as a separate entity.

Longitudinal fractures

These form perhaps 70 to 80 per cent of all temporal bone fractures and are usually the result of blows to the side of the head. The skin of the ear canal and eardrum are torn so that there is bleeding and sometimes a cerebrospinal fluid leak from the ear. This is such a strong sign that with the relevant history of injury, allows a diagnosis of a fracture to the base of the skull to be made in the absence of positive plain x-ray findings, which are difficult to interpret, at least as far as fractures are concerned. There is always involvement of the middle ear structures in this form of injury with disruption of the ossicles in the severest cases and consequently a conductive hearing loss. Fortunately,

Figure 6.2: Diagram of the base of the skull showing the path of a typical longitudinal fracture. The air spaces of the mastoid, middle ear and Eustachian tube are shaded and the internal carotid artery (ica) is cross-hatched. The other structures are: of, optic foramen; fr, foramen rotundum; fo, foramen ovale; fs, foramen spinosum; ips, inferior petrosal sinus; iam, internal auditory meatus; eac, external auditory canal; jf, jugular fossa; ss, sigmoid sinus; hc, hypoglossal (XII) canal; fm, foramen magnum. The fracture line is shown by the heavy zig-zag.

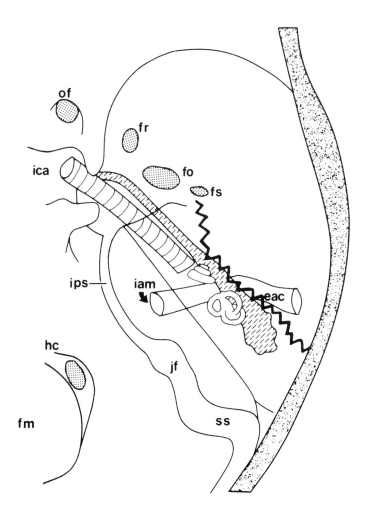

Figure 6.3: The more complex pathway of a transverse fracture of the temporal bone is shown, again by the heavy zig-zag line. Several fragments can be produced but the fracture line runs through the labyrinth. Annotation as for Figure 6.2.

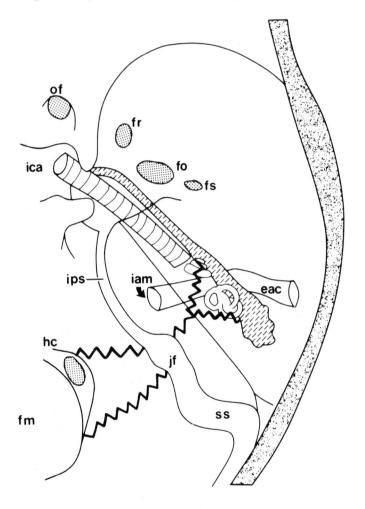

the fracture line does not run into the labyrinth so that major sensorineural deafness and vertigo are not a major feature of this injury. The presence of vertigo with nystagmus suggests other possibilities. There may be an additional transverse fracture when a sensorineural deafness is also present. There may have been trauma to the neck and brainstem when the nystagmus might not be typical of a labyrinthine lesion and there will be no major sensorineural deafness. Finally, trauma might have caused rupture of the round or oval windows when a sensorineural deafness is likely to be present. A pure sensorineural hearing loss, sometimes with tinnitus, can also occur with longitudinal fractures. In this case, as in those where there is no fracture present, the hearing loss tends to be for the higher frequencies and may improve with time. It is thought to be due to a shaking-up and limited physical disruption of the organ of Corti which is much more fragile than the vestibular portion of the labyrinth.

The facial nerve is involved in about 20 per cent of these fractures and as a general principle a facial palsy of immediate onset needs surgical exploration as soon as the patient is fit enough, whilst a palsy of delayed onset can be treated conservatively. The reason for mentioning this feature is to encourage you to record somewhere in the notes or hospital referral letter the state of the facial nerve when the patient was first seen. All that is needed is 'VII, OK' or 'VII complete palsy', as it makes the decisions about subsequent management so much easier if this piece of information is available.

Transverse fractures

These are thought to be the result of blows to the back of the head and account for about 20 per cent of all temporal bone fractures. There is no bleeding from the ear canal but blood can be seen behind the eardrum which is intact. Occasionally the bleeding is so profuse that blood is forced along the Eustachian tube to present in the mouth or nose. Since the labyrinth is disrupted there is a profound rotary vertigo and a vestibular-type horizontal nystagmus with a fast phase away from the injured side. Other types of nystagmus, especially a spontaneous vertical nystagmus, or a horizontal one that changes direction as the gaze is altered from side to side, suggests that something is happening centrally. The peripheral-type nystagmus will settle over a few days, and the patient will often not be troubled by vertigo after the first days or so as he is usually confined to bed. However, as soon as he tries to get up and about he is found to be unsteady and complains of 'dizziness'. This can persist for a long time depending upon the degree and speed of compensation, and sometimes the label 'post-concussional neurosis' is unfortunately donated by those unfamiliar with the problem.

107

Animal experimentation has shown that following a uni-lateral labyrinthectomy, the speed of recovery of normal balance is significantly reduced if the animal is restricted, rather than allowed to be freely mobile. The same presumably occurs in humans restricted by plaster casts and traction so that wher-ever possible physiotherapy should be arranged to provide improvised vestibular exercises.

There is, in addition, a profound sensorineural hearing loss which can confuse those who assume that the deafness is due to blood in the middle ear. A simple whisper and tuning fork test gives the correct answer, but unfortunately the deafness, unlike the vertigo, does not recover. A facial palsy is present in 50 per cent of transverse fractures and is frequently of immediate onset. This should be explored as soon as possible since long delay seems to worsen the chances of recovery.

As a general principle the presence of blood in the ear canal in the longitudinal fractures, or behind the eardrum in the transverse type means that the fracture is technically compound. There is therefore always the risk of an ascending infection causing a meningitis and no attempt should be made to clean out the ear canal. Antibiotics are also indicated in these patients, the exact combination depending on the prescribing practice of the doctor or local unit.

Concussion of the central vestibular pathways

Vertigo or vague unsteadiness following injury often has its origins outside the labyrinth. Animal studies have shown that in whiplash injuries, where the head is free and never strikes another object, patchy small bleeds and oedema occur in the brainstem and cerebellum. Following such injuries in man you can often see short-lived direction-changing nystagmus indica-tive of some central problem. In many patients the acute symp-toms of vertigo or unsteadiness, resulting from direct trauma without fracture or from whiplash injuries, settle quickly, pre-sumably as the oedema in the brainstem and cerebellum resolves. In others the symptoms persist and prolong convales-cence suggesting that there are small areas of damage and that central compensation is slow. On testing there may be a positional nystagmus with vertigo or unsteadiness that does not conform to the pattern of the classic benign positional nystagmus. Formal bithermal caloric tests can also reveal a partial canal paresis and a directional preponderance which further suggests central troubles. There may even be a psychological overlay prolonging recovery, and the involvement of a clutch of lawyers in matters of financial compensation seems only to make things worse.

The management is difficult with all these factors and in addition the possibility of bleeding and oedema in the labyrinth at the time of injury. In the early stages, vestibular sedatives are useful with strong reassurance that the symptoms will finally resolve. The early introduction of physiotherapy to the neck and a course of vestibular exercises seems to have some positive benefits, but sometimes in the elderly full recovery never comes and they can end up house-bound.

BAROTRAUMA

The perilymph is separated from the middle ear spaces by two membranes; the very thin round window membrane and the annular ligament around the stapes footplate. It also has a connection with the cerebrospinal fluid by way of a small canal running through the temporal bone called the cochlear aqueduct. Pressure applied to the perilymph can cause a rupture of one, or rarely both, of the membranes which either implode or explode depending on whether the raised pressure is external or internal. Whatever the route, the result is a leak of perilymph into the middle ear with a sensorineural hearing loss and vertigo. The size of the hole and the speed of the leak determine the magnitude of the deafness and dizziness and can cause problems in diagnosis when the symptoms are minor or intermittent. Raised intracranial pressure from direct closed head injury, free fall parachuting, and even apparently minor physical exertion during which a Valsalva manoeuvre is performed such as lifting a heavy object can cause the problem.

The cause may be obvious from the history but sometimes the symptoms are intermittent after lesser trauma and may not accompany the hearing loss which can itself be profound or fluctuating as occurs in Ménière's syndrome. Indeed, a perilymph leak may result in episodic bouts of vertigo which along with the fluctuating hearing loss makes differentiation from Ménière's disease very difficult if the history of trauma has been forgotten. Positional vertigo very much like the benign paroxysmal positional variety can arise but fail to settle as might be expected with the classic form. Finally, unsteadiness without vertigo is sometimes a troublesome complication and can arise spontaneously or after coughing and straining. Presumably, there is a very small leak of perilymph which is just enough to unsettle the vestibular labyrinth without pushing it over into an acute bout of vertigo.

The examination is usually unrewarding in that the eardrum is usually normal unless additional direct trauma has also occurred. The fistula test is occasionally positive and with a history of the trauma makes the diagnosis fairly certain. The audiogram will almost certainly show some sensorineural hearing loss which may be a high tone or flat. Positional tests sometimes produce a benign positional nystagmus with typical features, and a caloric test sometimes shows a partial canal paresis or a directional preponderance.

So far any diagnosis has been made on suspicion and very uncertain physical signs. The only way to confirm it is to inspect the two windows at operation. Clear-cut evidence of a leak even with the patient tilted head-down and with the jugular vein temporarily occluded is frequently lacking and often the diagnosis is made more in the hope of a happy outcome following repair rather than in response to what the surgeon sees. Nevertheless, in an established fistula covering the leak with fascia or fat after freshening up the surrounding mucosa usually stops the vertigo, although the chances of improving the hearing are slight.

Divers are also liable to inner ear problems as a complication of the bends when the nitrogen which, under great pressure, has been forced into the blood and some other tissues, comes out of solution as bubbles during decompression. This field of medicine is outside the scope of this book but Farmer (1977) is a good starting point.

7

Ménière's Syndrome

Prosper Ménière described an episodic, fluctuating but slowly progressive condition consisting of bouts of hearing loss and tinnitus associated with attacks of vertigo, which he ascribed to disease in the inner ear. Were he alive today he would probably be disappointed by the way his name has often been used as an indiscriminate label for various forms of dizziness that do not yield themselves to easy diagnosis. He might also be dismayed by the general lack of progress made in describing the pathology, in discovering the cause or producing an effective treatment for the condition that carries his name.

Part of the reason is that Ménière's syndrome is a fickle sort of complaint whose progress is measured in decades rather than years and which rarely kills the patient. It is not possible to biopsy the inner ear without destroying its function and well-preserved post-mortem specimens are rare. There is no specific diagnostic test for the disease, and it has proved impossible to find an animal model that even remotely resembles the clinical picture found in man.

PRESENTATION

Although there is a range of forms of presentation, most otologists feel that a tetrad of symptoms should be involved at some time during the course of the disease (Table 7.1). A diagnosis of Ménière's syndrome should be made when an underlying medical or surgical condition is discovered as Ménière's disease is, at least for the time being, idiopathic.

The most frequent form of presentation would be as likely in

111

Table 7.1: Criteria for diagnosing Ménière's syndrome

1. Episodic vertigo
2. Fluctuating unilateral or bilateral sensorineural hearing loss
3. Tinnitus in the affected ear or ears
4. A feeling of fullness in the ear

a male as in a female and they would most probably be in their thirties or forties. Onset in the first and last few decades of life is very uncommon. They could well have a job in which they feel, or on reflection felt, they were under pressure. The first symptoms, which could well be ignored, are usually auditory, with a soft, often low-pitched tinnitus appearing in one ear. This is frequently accompanied by a sense of fullness in the same ear. The two will disappear after a few days, often to be forgotten until some weeks, months and only rarely years later, when the sensations return perhaps this time associated with some hearing loss. This may be slight or severe but more remarkable is the distortion of the hearing that remains. This can bring about some peculiar descriptions as patients try to put into words the alterations of pitch, the prolongation of sounds and the abnormal loudness that can occur.

The symptoms fluctuate and may seem to disappear, in some cases for periods of many months. Sooner or later, however, the vestibular portion of the inner ear becomes involved, and the diagnosis of Ménière's syndrome becomes complete when vertigo develops. Morrison (1984) suggests that the full complex has developed within six months of the first remembered symptom in 60 per cent of his patients.

The first attack of vertigo must be a frightening experience, and the classic history comprises a recurrence of the fullness in the ear that may increase to a pulsating pain, a sudden increase in the intensity of the tinnitus, and if noticed a diminution of the hearing. Shortly after vertigo develops. This attack is not a momentary affair but a more severe disturbance lasting many minutes, hours or even up to a day. The intensity of the vertigo varies from very mild, with merely unsteadiness, to disastrous, when the patient is forced to the ground by the feeling of rotation. The attacks can occur at any time, even waking the patient from their sleep (and thereby distinguishing the disease from a psychogenic disorder). Depending on the susceptibility of the individual, there is associated nausea, pallor, sweating and vomiting, which may become the most distressing complaint.

Finally, the attack settles, the tinnitus is noticed to have diminished, the fullness in the ear has almost gone and the hearing has probably improved, but usually not quite to the level preceding the attack.

Sooner or later another attack occurs. It may be more or less intense, or of longer or shorter duration than the first. In general the attacks tend to cluster with active spells lasting for a few weeks or months, interspersed with quiescent spells lasting months or years. During these times there may be only an irritating tinnitus and distorted hearing.

As the years turn into decades the character of the disease tends to alter with the severity of the attacks of vertigo tending to diminish and the hearing loss, which is now quite severe, and the tinnitus tending to remain stable. Some cases appear to 'burn themselves out'. However, other disturbances of the vestibular part of the labyrinth may make an appearance and 'drop attacks' (Tumarkin 1936) can occur, although it is very difficult to be certain that these are the result of Ménière's disease rather than another pathology in the ageing patient. Chronic unsteadiness may develop with bouts of short-lived vertigo superimposed, turning the patient into a housebound, partly deafened, often depressed invalid. Occasionally the patient may develop a positional vertigo. This symptom, like the drop attacks might cause concern since brainstem disease is part of the differential diagnosis of positional vertigo. Finally, and especially if the disease started when the patient was in their teens or twenties, the other ear can become involved and the disease pattern recur, resulting in a severely deafened and unsteady individual.

The appearance of the various components of Ménière's disease is usually as described with unilateral hearing loss and tinnitus preceding the vertigo (Watanabe 1980). All three can occur simultaneously, but for episodic vertigo to be the sole complaint is unusual (Morrison 1975), and if it persists as the only symptom without any detectable hearing loss for a year, should prompt further investigation for there is almost certainly some other disease at work.

EXAMINATION

Most patients are probably seen between the acute attacks when there will be no signs of any spontaneous vestibular disorder. An examination of the ears will be normal. A full neurological examination will reveal no disorder of the cranial nerves except a loss of hearing on the affected side. There will usually be no signs of unsteadiness. Romberg's test will not reveal any tendency to topple one way or the other, provided there is no major psychological overlay. Tests of cerebellar function will reveal no ataxia, and the long tracts as tested by vibration sense will be normal. The blood pressure will be normal. In Ménière's syndrome some evidence of an underlying disorder may make an appearance.

During the attacks however, the relatives or doctor may notice nystagmus. In Ménière's disease any spontaneous nystagmus is nearly always that typical of a unilateral peripheral, vestibular failure with a horizontal nystagmus and a fast phase away from the affected ear. If the patient can co-operate during this time he will also tend to stagger or fall to the affected side. These signs rapidly disappear as the attack passes.

INVESTIGATIONS

There is no simple diagnostic test for Ménière's disease. The diagnosis is made from the history and the negative examination, apart from hearing loss, between the attacks. Investigations really serve to add weight to the diagnosis and, more importantly, to exclude other conditions. Blood disorders and diabetes must be ruled out. The tests to support the diagnosis fall into two groups; auditory and vestibular.

Auditory

Clinical

Whisper and tuning fork tests, provided adequate masking is used, reveal a unilateral sensorineural loss, in the majority of cases, where only one ear is involved.

Pure tone audiometry

Patients typically have a low tone, sensorineural loss in the early stages of the disease, but an additional high-pitched element can give an inverted V shape to the audiogram (Figure 7.1). On repeated testing the hearing, mainly in the low frequencies, may fluctuate from week to week, but as the years pass by, the audiogram tends to flatten out and perhaps a 60 dB sensori-neural hearing loss is recorded with little, if any, fluctuation detectable. In very longstanding disease there may be virtually no detectable hearing in the affected ear, but this is uncommon.

Test of recruitment

Recruitment occurs in early Ménière's disease. It can be detected audiometrically by Fowler's alternate binaural loud-ness balance test (Fowler 1950) (Figure 7.2) or by the thresholds for the stapedial reflex when the normal 70−80 dB gap between the pure tone threshold and reflex threshold is reduced (Figure 7.3). Additional tests are listed in Table 7.2 and are described further in the section on audiology in Chapter 19. In longstanding disease, and especially in those with profound deafness an element of neural loss becomes evident and some of the results will alter to suggest retrocochlear involvement. If the patient is seen for the first time at a late stage of the disease such finding may cause concern and further investigation.

Electric response audiometry

In Ménière's syndrome a typical but not diagnostic electro-cochleographic pattern is found. The waveform characteristic-ally shows an enhanced negative summating potential and the ratio of·the magnitude of this to the action potential, when the threshold is greater than 40 dB, is probably the firmest indicator of a diagnosis of Ménière's syndrome, provided syphilis has been excluded (Gibson, Prasher and Kilkenny 1983) (Figure 7.4). The brainstem responses are typically normal.

Vestibular

In the early stages of Ménière's disease the caloric test is usually within normal limits although the responses may even be hyper-active (Hart 1984). As the disease progresses, vestibular failure

115

Figure 7.1: Two audiograms showing bone conduction levels only for the right ear and indicating typical changes found in Ménière's disease.

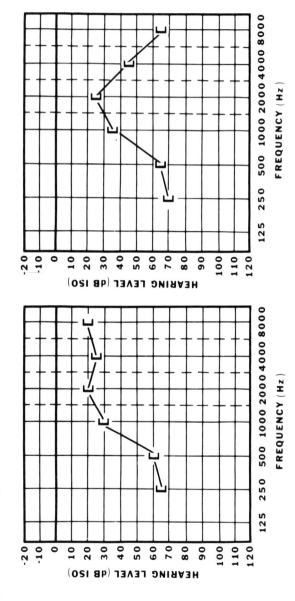

Figure 7.2: Fowler's alternate binaural loudness balance test. The boxes indicate the sound pressures that appear equally loud in the good and the bad ear. The approach of the test curve to the normal-45° dotted line indicates recruitment.

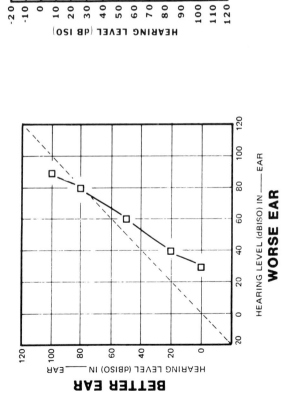

Figure 7.3: Stapedial reflex threshold in an ear with a sensorineural hearing loss that is showing recruitment. The normal 70–80 dB gap between the pure tone threshold and the stapedial reflex threshold has been reduced to 35–40 dB in this case.

C Stapedial reflex threshold

Table 7.2: Summary of audiometric tests in Ménière's syndrome

Test	Result
Pure tone	Sensorineural loss
Alternate binaural loudness balance	Recruiting
Stapedial reflex	Recruiting: no decay
Bekesy	Type 2 or 4
Tone decay	0–25 dB
Sort increment sensitivity index	Positive
Tympanometry	Normal
Electrocochleography	Enhanced summating potential

becomes apparent as a canal paresis, although this is not usually complete. A profound canal paresis should suggest some other destructive lesion of the inner ear or vestibular nerve.

DIFFERENTIAL DIAGNOSIS

Many conditions may mimic some aspects of Ménière's disease. Isolated vestibular symptoms without any localising signs are frequently labelled as Ménière's disease without any evidence for the other criteria of the condition. Perhaps the unsatisfactory diagnosis of vertigo of unknown cause should be made more often, after a thorough examination, and time allowed to pass for the condition to resolve spontaneously or to declare itself as other symptoms and signs evolve. Conditions that can be mistaken for Ménière's disease are listed in Table 7.3 with late syphilis being foremost.

INCIDENCE

With incomplete agreement as to what makes a positive diagnosis of Ménière's disease, and the frequent need for long-term assessment before a diagnosis can be made, it is not surprising that figures for the incidence vary (Table 7.4). Similar problems relate to the assessment of the occurrence of bilateral disease. Greven and Oosterveld (1975) reported that depending on the

Table 7.3: Differential diagnosis of Ménière's syndrome

Treponemal disease:	late syphilis
	congenital syphilis
	yaws
Middle ear disease, especially cholesteatoma	
Otosclerosis and Paget's disease	
Delayed endolymphatic hydrops following:	labyrinthitis
	meningitis
	sudden deafness of viral origin
Acoustic neuroma	
Multiple sclerosis	
Basilar migraine	

Table 7.4: Incidence of Ménière's syndrome in white Caucasians

Place	Author	Annual incidence in population (%)
Northern Ireland	Wilmot (1979)	0.01 – 0.02
Sweden	Stahle et al. (1978)	0.046
Wales	Griffiths (1979)	0.1
Britain	Hinchcliffe (1961)	1.1

Figure 7.4: Typical electrocochleographic recordings from a normal ear and a Ménière's ear when loud sounds are used for testing. The negative summating potential which just precedes the whole nerve action potential is enhanced in Ménière's cases and the waveform of the action potential is grossly widened.

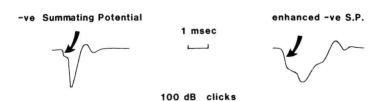

Normal   **Ménière's**

-ve Summating Potential   enhanced -ve S.P.

1 msec

100 dB clicks

strictness of the diagnostic criteria, the second ear could be said to be involved in between 10 and 70 per cent of their patients.

119

AETIOLOGY

It is also not surprising that the cause of Ménière's disease is unknown since the physiology of the normal inner ear is still not understood. The mechanism of the origin and maintenance of endolymph is obscure as is the mechanism of the cochlea's ability to discriminate pitch. Histopathological findings from the temporal bones of patients with Ménière's disease frequently show dilatation of the membranous labyrinth. This change, however, appears to be non-specific occurring in syphilitic ear disease, other longstanding inner ear disease, sometimes in apparently normal ears, and also in poorly preserved material. Nevertheless the weight of evidence suggests that some malfunction of endolymph homeostasis occurs, and may result in small fluctuating pressure changes within the membranous labyrinth. The cochlea at least is remarkably sensitive to pressure changes, with minute fluctuations severely reducing the ability of the organ of Corti to detect pitch and intensity.

The endolymphatic sac (Figure 7.5), an appendage to the membranous labyrinth has been thought to play some role in the turnover of the endolymph by active resorption. It is highly vascularised and alterations in its blood supply may well affect its function and consequently that of the cochlear and vestibular labyrinth. There are many conditions that can affect the micro-circulation, and may result in Ménière's syndrome. Disorders of the brainstem circulation from basilar artery disease, hypertension, excessive nicotine, obesity and diabetes are all candidates. There has been a strong argument developed for a psychosomatic element in the condition with Stephens (1975) reviewing previously published work and adding his own series. Together these suggest a marked preponderance of obsessional personality traits in the Ménière's group. The results of properly controlled trials of treatment confirm the importance of the psyche in the disease and its management.

Figure 7.5: Surgeon's view of the endolymphatic sac during a cortical mastoidectomy. The endolymphatic sac arises from a duct joining the utricle to saccule (see Figure 1.?) and passes inwards to lie between the bone and dura of the posterior cranial fossa.

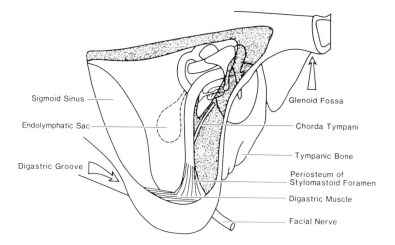

Sigmoid Sinus

Endolymphatic Sac

Digastric Groove

Glenoid Fossa

Chorda Tympani

Tympanic Bone

Periosteum of Stylomastoid Foramen

Digastric Muscle

Facial Nerve

TREATMENT

Treatment is made difficult by not knowing what causes the disease. Assessment of the results of treatment is made even harder by the lack of uniform diagnostic criteria, by the fluctuating nature and protracted course of the disease, and by the strong psychosomatic element, whereby any treatment enthusiastically offered brings relief to many. Consequently there are few guidelines to the optimum treatment especially in the intermediate stages of the disease.

However, in the early stages, especially when there is fluctuating hearing loss, firm medical management is often adequate. This includes taking time in explanation and reassurance that there is no sinister disease, and if you believe that 'stress' forms part of the cause, suggesting changes in the patient's lifestyle where appropriate. Abstinence from smoking should anyhow be encouraged most strongly. Many clinicians feel that restricting the amount of tea and coffee consumed may also help. Vestibular sedatives are useful during the active phase of the disease and as a long-term measure betahistine, a vaso-active drug, has

121

been found to be better than placebo in controlling many of the symptoms, if not in improving objective measurements of hearing and balance (Wilmot and Menon 1976). A cautious optimism should be conveyed to the patient and conscientious follow-up, preferably with the same doctor arranged. Wilmot (1979) believes that many patients seen early enough have reversible disease, but all too often the patient is first seen with established hearing loss and sometimes disabling bouts of vertigo. Some will manage well on medical treatment and can be continued on this for a long time. Many, because of the depression that frequently results from the miserable symptoms, will be helped with antidepressants. Others, because of the severity of the vertigo will be candidates for a surgical procedure.

A whole range of surgical procedures has evolved over the years. Many operations have been discarded as time has shown their ineffectiveness.

Those that have stood the test of time fall into two groups; conservative, where there is still serviceable hearing, and destructive, when the malfunctioning labyrinth is destroyed.

The endolymphatic sac is surgically accessible, with negligible risk of damage to the hearing, and may play some part in the evolution of the disease. Various manoeuvres to expose, incise or drain the sac have been devised and surprisingly, all have good early success rates with about 70 per cent cure or improvement of the vertigo at one year. The development of these procedures has been based on animal experiments where ligation or ablation of the sac results in the accumulation of endolymph. The anatomy of the endolymphatic sac in man is, however, quite different from that in most experimental animals (Lundquist, Rask-Andersen, Galey and Bagger-Sjöbäck 1984) and it has been suggested that the real effect of the operation is to alter the blood flow to the endolymphatic sac (Morrison 1984). However, a study by Thomsen, Bretlau, Tos and Johnsen (1981) compared the effects of an endolymphatic sac operation with a sham operation (a cortical mastoidectomy) in a carefully controlled trial that would probably no longer be feasible because of the Helsinki declaration on medical ethics. At one year there was little difference between the treatment and placebo operations, both groups having marked improvement in the vertigo, nausea and vomiting. This profound placebo effect will probably also account for the apparent success of inserting a ventilation tube (grommet) into the tympanic membrane, a procedure which is highly unlikely to have any direct effect on Ménière's disease. Nevertheless, surgery of the endolymphatic sac does seem to offer real symptomatic relief to many patients whatever the exact mechanism, and is probably first-line surgical treatment when there is still hearing.

In patients with no serviceable hearing and disabling vertigo, a labyrinthectomy will frequently provide complete relief from the vertigo if all the sensory epithelium is destroyed but may leave the older patient unsteady for a long time. This procedure is not always as successful as anticipated and this may well be due to intact post-ganglionic fibres in the vestibular nerve. A vestibular neurectomy will provide relief of vertigo in virtually all cases. If there is serviceable hearing, a middle cranial fossa approach dividing the nerve in the internal auditory meatus is an excellent operation, tolerated well in the young patient, that preserves the hearing with little risk of damage in the facial nerve. Where there is no useful hearing, the vestibular nerve can be divided by a translabyrinthine approach in which a labyrinthectomy is performed by way of approach to the internal auditory meatus. This provides effective relief from the vertigo, although again older patients may still be unsteady.

The recurrence of vertigo following a correctly performed labyrinthectomy or neurectomy is distressing to the patient and a dilemma to the surgeon as it suggests involvement of the other ear. If confirmed, preservation of hearing becomes the goal and conservative procedures the means. Improvements in otological, neurosurgical and anaesthetic skills have made vestibular neurectomy a realistic proposition in specialised centres and it should be seriously considered for those patients with disabling vertigo.

8

Paroxysmal Positional Vertigo

Benign paroxysmal positional vertigo (BPPV) is a common presentation of episodic dizziness. It usually arises without other ear symptoms but sometimes occurs during the course of acute or chronic otitis media, when the distinction from a serous labyrinthitis may be difficult. Occasionally burnt out or quiescent middle ear disease or Ménière's disease may precede the condition, but in the vast majority of cases there has either been some trauma to the head or an earlier viral upper respiratory tract infection.

Whatever the association, the presenting symptoms are precisely the same and are thought to arise from the debris formed during the degeneration of the otoconia of the utricle finding its way into the ampulla of the posterior semicircular canal and causing abnormal stimulation of the sensory cells in certain positions.

The first attack comes as a surprise, and it may be some time before it is realised that one particular head movement or change of position causes the momentary rotary vertigo as described in Chapter 2. This vertigo lasts for seconds or possibly minutes, but may be severe enough to make the patient stagger, feel sick and sometimes vomit. After a while it becomes apparent that the rapidity of head movement induces a more severe attack so that the neck is held stiffly and the patient is unwilling to move quickly.

BPPV disappears in the vast majority of patients within a few months and rarely persists beyond six. Even in those few in whom the symptoms continue, the vertigo may not be severe enough to disturb them excessively and they often learn to live with the complaint, or avoid the positional change that induces the trouble.

Following head injury the symptoms usually come on within a few days. In general the intensity and duration of the attacks is related to the severity of the injury but in the elderly especially quite a minor incident might be enough to cause the problem. Indeed, major symptoms resulting from what might have been minor trauma used to form part of a 'post-concussional neurosis' syndrome that was thought to be due to a personality defect or an attempt at malingering whether for financial compensation or attention. Although this might be the case in a few patients the vertigo itself is more likely to be the cause of the neurosis as it is particularly distressing and often provokes fears of something terrible going on inside the head.

Sometimes in the non-traumatic cases the episode of positional vertigo settles as expected after a few months, only to recur a year or so later, again to settle slowly. No satisfactory explanation for this clinical observation has ever been forthcoming.

The diagnosis is usually obvious on taking the history but I feel that it is important to perform the positional tests for induced nystagmus, as described in Chapter 3, for two reasons. First, it seems to give the patients a great sense of relief to know that the doctor can reproduce the symptoms exactly and can then explain that the condition is not harmful and will almost certainly go away of its own accord. Second, you must be sure that this condition is indeed benign as shown by the latency, duration, adaptation and fatigue of the induced nystagmus. Very occasionally brainstem disease will make its appearance as a positional vertigo and any deviation from the pattern of the benign response on positional testing means a complete neurological examination and probably referral to a neurologist. You should also examine the ears for evidence of middle ear disease, treat active otitis media and refer to an ENT surgeon if there is any suspicion of more serious trouble.

In the vast majority of sufferers the condition needs no active treatment other than examination, reassurance and a follow-up appointment. However, a few patients with severe, persisting BPPV may require surgical management with either destruction or disconnection of the malfunctioning labyrinth. If there is no useful hearing from old middle or inner ear disease then a labyrinthectomy will suffice. If serviceable hearing remains then some form of vestibular neurectomy is advisable. Gacek has long maintained that division of the nerve supplying the ampulla of the posterior semicircular canal is enough to solve the problem and this is certainly a less extensive operation than a middle cranial fossa vestibular neurectomy, although technically difficult and not without risks (Gacek 1983).

9

Vestibular Neuronitis and the Ramsay-Hunt Syndrome

The labyrinth, its nerve and nuclei, are sometimes involved in viral infections. A range of symptoms and signs results depending on which portions are involved and this feature has given rise to several named syndromes. Pure involvement of the vestibular portion has been called vestibular neuronitis, epidemic vertigo and neurolabyrinthitis amongst many other terms, and as is true in many branches of medicine, a variety of names usually means that the cause or pathology is obscure. Involvement of the cochlear portion results in a pure sensorineural hearing loss whilst the facial nerve can also be affected with a partial or complete facial palsy. Overlap sometimes occurs and the Ramsay-Hunt syndrome comprises a lower motor neurone facial palsy with, usually, a sensorineural deafness and vertigo. The herpes virus is the cause of this last syndrome, and could probably be incriminated in many cases of the other conditions although the mumps, measles and rubella viruses are also candidates as judged on a retrospective basis by changes in the specific antibody titres.

In pure vestibular neuronitis the site of damage appears to be the vestibular nerve where degenerative changes consistent with viral infection have been found in the very few specimens that have become available over the years.

The clinical picture is remarkably consistent in this condition with those in the age range 30 to 50 being most commonly involved. Nearly always a viral upper respiratory tract infection heralds the start of the troubles, with malaise, perhaps a low-grade fever and muscle aches and weakness being present. After a few days, often as these symptoms are subsiding, vertigo develops. The patient is at first unsteady but rapidly a profound vertigo arises which completely prostrates the individual and is usually, but not always, associated with nausea and vomiting. All the poor wretch can do is crawl to his bed where he lies quiet and still, feeling that the end of the world is nigh. The vertigo is usually rotary and persists for several days, indicating that the lesion is not entirely peripheral since central compensation would rapidly suppress trouble in the labyrinth. After a few days the patient finds he is able to move cautiously in bed, although rapid movement brings on the vertigo again. Gradually the troubles settle and he is able to get up, only to find that he is very unsteady, has difficulty walking and develops vertigo if he turns his head rapidly. Finally, the balance corrects itself, perhaps after a month or so, although in the elderly this may never be achieved. There are other forms of presentation either without the preceding viral infection, or, less commonly, with an insidious development of marked unsteadiness but without vertigo.

When seen during the acute vertiginous phase the patient is a pitiful sight and usually has a spontaneous horizontal or rotary nystagmus. The ears are normal, and there is no evidence of any hearing loss. The other cranial nerves, if you can test them, are intact. Often the patient is not seen until he has regained the use of his legs. He walks carefully, holding onto nearby objects and tends to keep his head still so that eye or body movement rather than head movement is used to look around. There is now no spontaneous nystagmus but eye movements are not quite right, and your finger is followed in a slightly jerky irregular fashion. The eyes come to rest at the lateral gaze position with a short wobble that could be mistaken for a vestibular type nystagmus but is not on closer observation.

Romberg's test, as described in Chapter 4, is negative in that there is no marked increase sway when the patient is standing and closes his eyes for two or three seconds. Caloric testing for induced nystagmus uniformly shows an absent or severely diminished response in one or both ears. A cool caloric is usually enough to make the diagnosis of absent canal function as a lack of response on this test is virtually always confirmed by the more involved bithermal calorics which use a lesser stimulus.

The natural history of the disease is for complete spontaneous resolution after a short, stormy course. Recurrences are rare, but occasionally, twenty or thirty years after the initial attack, and with advancing age there may be general disturbances of balance with unsteadiness on rapid movement in someone who had never suffered like this in the intervening years. Presumably, the ageing vestibular system without adequate information from the labyrinth is unable to cope with the stress of unusual movement.

Unfortunately, there is a differential diagnosis for vestibular neuronitis, as disseminated sclerosis may present with, or have as part of its unfolding story, an attack that cannot be distinguished from the classic features of viral infection of the vestibular nerve. The only difference may be the absence of the prior upper respiratory tract infection, which anyhow is not mandatory for the diagnosis of vestibular neuronitis. Only a history of some other fleeting neurological disorder, or the passage of time, will allow the distinction to be made.

Management of the acute features of vestibular neuronitis or of a similar attack provoked by disseminated sclerosis rests on the administration of vestibular sedatives which usually need to be given intramuscularly because of the sickness, and reassurance that the world is not coming to an end. If complete recovery of balance is slow, the provision of vestibular exercises as described in Chapter 18 is sometimes helpful.

The Ramsay-Hunt syndrome also starts with a generalised malaise but this is rapidly followed by the onset of severe pain in or around the ear and then after a few days the eruption of a vesiculating rash on the outer surface of the external ear (Figure 9.1). Occasionally the vesicles are behind the ear and sometimes on the borders of the soft palate and tongue where the initial pain is also located. Sir William Osler once remarked that the man who could confidently diagnose shingles before the eruption of the rash knew all there was to know about medicine. This is especially true for the Ramsay-Hunt syndrome which is another expression of a herpes virus infection. As the rash develops, or more usually shortly after, a facial weakness develops on the same side. This can be partial but is nearly always complete and profound.

Deafness, tinnitus and vertigo usually make an appearance within another few days. The vertigo is frequently the most disabling part of the condition which is more common in the elderly, who may be especially bothered by the unsteadiness that persists after the vertigo has settled, which it usually does within a week.

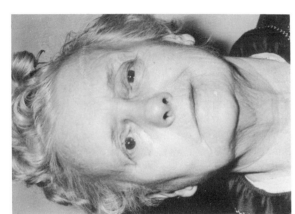

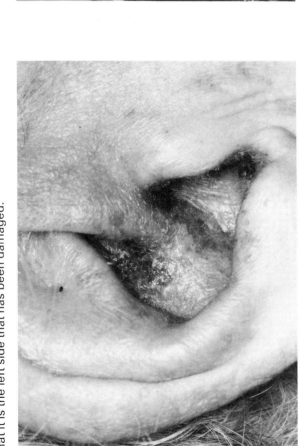

Figure 9.1: **(a)** Vesicles and crusting typical of the herpes virus infection causing a Ramsay-Hunt syndrome. This patient, an elderly lady presented with a facial palsy, vertigo and a sensorineural deafness. The vesicles erupted a day after the other symptoms. **(b)** Facial view of the patient attempting to smile and thereby revealing the typical features of a right-sided palsy. The face looks distorted on her left and it is easy to make the mistake of thinking that it is the left side that has been damaged.

Early on, an examination reveals the rash, which occasionally can be seen deep in the ear canals, the facial palsy and the sensorineural deafness. Spontaneous vestibular-type horizontal nystagmus is usually present with the fast phase away from the affected side. It is initially seen in all directions of gaze (third, second and first degree) but rapidly settles to a first degree nystagmus which soon fades. Sometimes the vertigo is slight from the onset with only a first degree nystagmus and the cochlear deafness can be minor and reversible. The facial nerve, however, is very slow to recover and frequently never does, so that problems of corneal irritation can arise because of the inability to close the eye.

Management in the early stages requires analgesics and vestibular sedatives, but the disabling unsteadiness that can arise in the long-term in the elderly may be helped by vestibular exercises.

10

Syphilitic Ear Disease

Unfortunately syphilis is not that uncommon a disease and can present with vertigo or unsteadiness usually associated with deafness and tinnitus so that it may often be confused with a whole host of other conditions. Dunlop (1972) reports that in the 25 years from 1946 there were 178,000 cases of acquired and congenital syphilis in England and Wales, and there is growing evidence that, once established, syphilitic ear disease never completely resolves however well it is treated. The best that can be hoped for is for a halt in its otherwise relentless progression.

The unsteadiness that results from syphilis may be caused by expression of the disease elsewhere than in the temporal bone. Loss of input from the somatosensors because of damage to the posterior columns of the spinal cord or even gradual failure of vision from ocular involvement are both possible. Syphilis will therefore crop up again in the remainder of this book, so that a brief review of its natural history is presented here. The disease can be congenital or acquired and the course of untreated acquired syphilis is conveniently and conventionally separated into three stages.

ACQUIRED SYPHILIS

Primary stage

Ten days to ten weeks after transfer of the spirochaete, *Treponema pallidum*, the primary lesion, the chancre, appears on the involved skin or mucosa. This is usually the genitals but may be on the lips, in the mouth, in or around the anus or on a finger. A thickened clear, usually painless ulcer develops with soft firm painless enlargement of the local lymph nodes. This enlargement seems disproportionately great compared to the rather harmless looking ulcer. Primary lesions heal spontaneously within a few weeks.

Secondary stage

From the third to the sixth month, evidence of generalised infection becomes apparent in most patients by the development of skin lesions. These are frequently asymptomatic in that they may not bother the individual enough to warrant a trip to the doctor. A description of all the different skin conditions would probably fill half a dermatology text book, but there are four cardinal signs of the secondary stage:

1. Cutaneous rashes: these are the most common and the early rash is a faint, reddish flat discoloration (macular erythema) that may spread and later becomes darker in colour. A papular erythema comprises rather more discrete reddish raised lesions that, like the macular form are present over all the body or may be restricted to a small area. Both rashes may be found on the hands but neither of them is itchy;
2. Condylomata: on the anus or around the genitalia, small eroded heaped up moist papules may be present and can resemble warts. They are termed condylomata lata, contain spirochaetes and are highly infective;
3. Snail track ulcers: on the mucous membranes of the mouth and pharynx, oval, round or arcuate patches develop and may ulcerate to form shallow tracks with a reddish edge and a central off-white slough. They are also highly infective;
4. Lymphadenopathy: generalised painless lymphadenopathy forms the fourth cardinal symptom or sign of the secondary syphilis.

In addition, the patient may have a headache, sore throat, a generalised malaise and a low irregular fever. At this stage of the disease one-third of patients have changes detectable in the cerebrospinal fluid, indicating central nervous system involvement, and a few will develop meningitis with involvement of some of the cranial nerves, but predominantly the VIII nerve. These features generally last between three weeks and three months although perhaps a quarter of patients will have later relapses.

Tertiary or late syphilis

Following the secondary lesions an untreated patient enters a latent period without symptoms or signs. This will last from two to thirty years as the spirochaetes, which have been disseminated throughout the body remain quiescent as latent syphilis. However, the interplay between the spirochaete and the host's immunity may alter and an enormous range of local complications may arise; as neurosyphilis in one-third, cardiovascular syphilis in another third or benign tertiary syphilis in a final third. Rarely visceral syphilis can occur. Alternatively, the disease can slowly be eradicated by the immune system so that a spontaneous cure arises (Knox, Musher and Guzick, 1976) (Figure 10.1).

CONGENITAL SYPHILIS

Congenital syphilis results from transplacental infection after the fourth month of gestation and may result in stillbirth. If a live birth results, the symptoms of congenital syphilis can be present in the newborn child when they are fulminating or develop in later life. There are a whole range of manifestations of congenital syphilis with perhaps more than one-third developing a sensorineural hearing loss (Karmody and Schuknecht 1966) in addition to a variable expression of the other features that will also be present. Table 10.1 indicates in descending order the features most likely to be present when there is involvement of the VIII nerve.

VERTIGO AND SYPHILIS

Although vertigo is more commonly found in cases of late and congenital disease it can very occasionally arise during the

Figure 10.1: Highly schematic diagram of the possible outcomes of syphilis. There is a continuing interplay between the virulence of the organism and the patient's immunity so that any individual may or may not show symptoms depending on the exact balance. Some never manifest late symptoms and remain as latent syphilitics whilst others seem to undergo spontaneous cure.

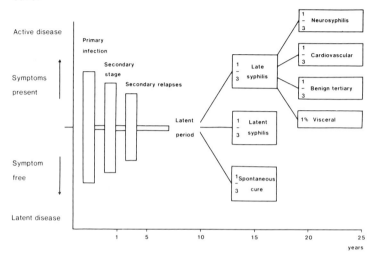

Source: After Knox *et al.* (1976).

Table 10.1: Manifestations of congenital syphilis. Those most commonly associated with deafness are near the top of the table

Hutchinson's triad: Hutchinson's peg-teeth
                  Interstitial keratitis of the cornea
                  VIIIN deafness
Bossing of the frontal bones
Saddle nose
Fissures at the angles of the mouth (Rhagades)
Clutton's joints
High arched palate
Short maxilla
Sabre tibia
Skin lesions
In children:
    Mucopurulent rhinitis
    Splenomegaly
    Anaemia
Generalised lymphadenopathy

135

secondary stage even though treatment has apparently been adequate. The majority of the few cases that have been recognised present with an acute rotary vertigo with its associated nausea and vomiting. There is usually an associated headache and may even be a slight fever so that in the absence of any hearing loss the diagnosis of a viral vestibular neuronitis is incorrectly made. More often, there is an additional sensorineural hearing loss that is usually bilateral and is frequently rapidly progressive when a diagnosis of 'labyrinthitis' may be made. In the studies where caloric testing was performed a canal paresis was present in all of the patients who complained of vertigo (Vercoe 1976; Balkany and Dans 1978).

It seems that aggressive treatment with a penicillin or cephalosporin following an initial dose of a steroid, to reduce the chances of a Herxheimer reaction, can be successful in settling the vertigo and in improving the hearing.

Most cases of vertigo, however, arise in the late acquired or congenital forms of the disease, and although the problem is not great in terms of the number of patients involved it is important in that the vertigo can often be improved. The accompanying hearing loss is, without treatment, relentlessly progressive, and is one of the few types of sensorineural hearing loss that can be altered by treatment so that diagnosis is not just academic.

In Morrison's study of syphilitic deafness, a work well worth reading, vestibular symptoms were found in association with the hearing loss in three-quarters of those with a congenital loss and in a half of those with a late acquired loss (Morrison 1975). The vestibular symptoms usually arise at the same time as the deafness although there is sometimes a gap of a few years with the deafness coming first. The symptoms of vestibular failure fall into two approximately equal groups.

Episodic vertigo

Prolonged bouts of rotary vertigo indicating acute changes within the labyrinth can occur. They last for many minutes or even up to a day or two. Nausea and vomiting are usually associated, and if syphilis is not considered, a whole range of diagnoses can result depending on whether the additional hearing loss, which may not be severe, is noticed by the patient or the doctor. In many patients the history cannot be distinguished from that of Ménière's disease, and indeed the only feature that allows separation is the positive serological findings in syphilis.

Unsteadiness

In this group, a slow, smooth, progressive destruction of both labyrinths results in increasing unsteadiness especially in the dark and when visual input is reduced. Many patients have additional corneal opacities and partial blindness and can be severely disabled.

The caloric tests in nearly all patients of both groups will be abnormal showing a profound loss of vestibular function in those with gross unsteadiness and those with longstanding bouts of vertigo. Morrison also notes that even in those with deafness but without vestibular symptoms the caloric tests were abnormal in half the patients, suggesting that the proposed slow, asymptomatic destruction of the vestibular labyrinth was taking place.

The diagnosis of syphilis is made first by thinking of the condition and then sending blood for serology. In the late acquired group, symptoms rarely commence before the age of 35 years whilst they can present at any time in the congenital group although the peak incidence is between the ages of 20 and 50 years. A history of acquired syphilis is often forgotten, suppressed or may not even have been considered if the primary and secondary stages were neglected or inadvertently treated with only a short course of perhaps an inappropriate antibiotic. Even in those adequately treated with multiple courses of penicillin, VIII nerve symptoms can still arise through spirochaetes lying dormant in the temporal bone and out of reach of the antibiotic. There may be no other stigmata of late syphilis although in the congenital group corneal opacities from old interstitial keratitis are common, and bear referral to an ophthalmologist if this has not already been done.

The examination will reveal a sensorineural hearing loss that can be of virtually any type; high tone, low tone, flat or peaked. Both ears are usually equally affected although in 20 per cent there is asymmetry in the level of the audiogram in the two ears. On more sophisticated testing, the deafness is usually cochlear in origin although in the profoundly deaf a neural element creeps in to confuse the results (see Glossary, Chapter 19).

Caloric testing will reveal some form of abnormality ranging from partial vestibular failure in one ear, usually the deafer one, to complete bilaterally absent responses. It is also important to test the vibration senses in the feet and legs as there may be changes which will make management of the unsteadiness all the more difficult.

The single most reliable diagnostic test is the Fluorescent Treponemal Antibody-Absorbed Test (FTA-Abs) performed on a sample of serum. This very rarely gives a false negative group and then only in the congenital group. You should specify this test when you fill in the request form.

Management of syphilitic ear disease

This really is a problem, and discussion as to the best method fills many a book and journal. The problem has many facets.

1. Spirochaetes lie sequestered in the temporal bone even after large doses of antisyphilitic treatment;
2. Penicillin is effective only when the organism is dividing, but in late syphilis the rate of division is very slow, maybe once every 90 days (Lawton-Smith 1969);
3. Giving steroids has several effects: it may encourage the spirochaetes to divide, but also protects against damage caused by a local inflammatory response.

A plan for treatment could therefore look something like this:

1. Start with a loading dose of a steroid and continue this at a reduced level during subsequent antibiotic treatment;
2. Add large doses of intramuscular penicillin for at least ten days, with oral probenecid to lower excretion of the penicillin and raise blood levels;
3. Continue oral steroids in a reducing dose to 5 mg prednisolone per day for one month;
4. If the audiogram improves or the vertigo resolves continue on a maintenance dose of steroids and repeat the course of intramuscular penicillin at, say, six months or a year;
5. If there is no improvement at all at the end of the month then withdraw the steroids;
6. Steroids may need to be continued at maintenance levels to

abolish the vertigo, but intermittent annual courses of intramuscular penicillin should then be given;

7. If there are allergic reactions to penicillin, a cephalosporin should be used although there is still a small group who will be cross-sensitive.

For dosage schedules, McNulty and Fassett (1981) or Morrison (1975), should be consulted.

The management of those who are unsteady because of loss of labyrinthine function is more difficult. If there is any useful hearing then a steroid and penicillin regimen should be started since untreated there is a relentless progression to profound deafness. Everything possible should be done to maintain optimum eyesight. The provision of a walking stick to add extra somatosensory input through the hands and arms is a simple and often very effective remedy.

11

Miscellaneous Ear Conditions

WAX

Surprisingly a lump of wax impacted in the depths of the ear canal and lying on the eardrum can produce unsteadiness and sometimes bouts of vertigo. These complaints seem to arise more frequently after the patient has been swimming or has otherwise managed to get water in the ear, when the wax swells and presumably distorts the eardrum and the ossicular chain thereby transferring the pressure change to the inner ear. If the wax completely occludes the canal there will also be a conductive deafness.

The diagnosis in this patient will be fairly obvious although the treatment may sometimes cause problems.

Syringing the wax is a time-honoured procedure that usually works. There is often a fear of perforating the eardrum by the force of the stream of water, but using cadavers it has been shown that the normal eardrum does not rupture under even quite forceful streams of water. Previous perforation or old scars on the eardrum are more fragile however, and you should be reluctant to syringe an ear if there is a history of perforation or if there is a mucoid discharge from the ear, for this means that there is certainly a hole in the eardrum.

The general idea behind syringing wax is to run a stream of water very close to body temperature along the roof of the ear canal so that it gets behind the wax and pushes it out along the canal. If the wax is rock hard or completely occludes the canal this can be difficult so it is wise to soften up the wax beforehand. The most effective agent is a mixture of sodium bicarbonate, glycerol and water. Olive oil is nearly as good. Either preparation should not come straight from the fridge as, not only can the experience be painful, but a caloric vertigo and nystagmus might be induced. The instructions in the British National Formulary are perfect — 'The patient should lie with the affected ear uppermost for 5 to 10 minutes after a generous amount of the solution has been introduced into the ear'. This should be repeated on 3 or 4 days prior to syringing. There are a whole host of proprietary wax solvents on the market. Many contain organic solvents which frequently irritate the canal skin and cause an otitis externa and if there is a perforation cause a remarkably intense pain if they get into the middle ear. Would you put paradichlorobenzine or turpentine oil in your middle ear?

If these attempts have been unsuccessful you may have to refer the patient to an ENT clinic for removal of the wax by suction with the aid of a good light and magnification provided by an operating microscope.

OTOSCLEROSIS

As well as the vertigo that can result from the surgery of otosclerosis (Chapter 7) the disease itself can also cause problems. Classic otosclerosis presents as a conductive hearing loss secondary to an overgrowth of bone around the anterior portion of the footplate of the stapes. This new bone formation is at first spongy — hence the French term otiospongiosus — and it is due to active bone resorption occurring at the same time as new bone is being laid down nearby. Calcification subsequently occurs but the new mass of bone is never harder than the original so that the term otosclerosis is a misnomer that has stuck in the literature. The mobility of the footplate decreases until it is finally fixed and unable to transmit pressure changes to the perilymph. The condition tends to be familial, occurring especially in females and the growth of the new bone is probably speeded up by pregnancy and the contraceptive pill. The diagnosis is usually fairly simple with a history of a slowly progressive hearing loss affecting one ear first and the other soon after, a normal eardrum on examination, and a conductive loss on tuning fork tests. Audiometry confirms the conductive nature of the hearing loss and stapedial reflexes are absent. (See Glossary, Chapter 19, for further information about the stapedial reflexes.) The diagnosis can be confirmed at operation by elevating the eardrum and finding that the stapes is not mobile.

Treatment is with a hearing aid — this is the sort of deafness that is best helped by simple amplification of sound — or by a stapedectomy. In this procedure the stapes is removed and the otosclerotic focus is by-passed using some sort of prosthesis between the long process of the incus and the perilymph.

The pathology that causes the stapes fixation can also arise at other sites in the bony labyrinth and cause both a sensorineural deafness, sometimes associated with tinnitus, and vertigo. How the otosclerosis causes these problems is not known, although there are strong arguments for changes in various enzyme levels in the perilymph being the culprit (Causse, Shambaugh, Causse and Bretlau 1980).

The dizziness that results from involvement of the vestibular part of the labyrinth comes in three forms (Cody and Baker 1978):

1. Spontaneous recurrent attacks of either vertigo or severe unsteadiness without the illusion of movement. The attacks can occur every day or infrequently and with the associated hearing loss, tinnitus, nausea and vomiting resemble Ménière's disease, so much so that cochlear otosclerosis forms part of the differential diagnosis of this condition. These spontaneous recurrent attacks are the most common vestibular symptom;

2. Postural vertigo or unsteadiness lasting for a few minutes, and brought on by rapid changes in the position of the head or movement of the body. Transient nausea is common but vomiting not;

3. A single spontaneous episode of vertigo or unsteadiness is the least common form of presentation. The attack lasts hours, days or even up to three weeks and is associated with nausea and vomiting so that symptoms rather like vestibular neuronitis develop except that there is an associated hearing loss.

In general, the symptoms are more severe the worse the hearing loss. The caloric responses will usually be depressed or even absent and the magnitude of the loss of vestibular response mirrors the sensorineural hearing loss.

The diagnosis of cochlear otosclerosis with vestibular symptoms rests on the following principles (Shambaugh and Holder-man 1926):

1. A family history of stapedial otosclerosis;
2. Bilateral symmetric sensorineural hearing loss, with one ear having a fixed stapes;
3. A sensorineural loss that has unusual audiometric configur-ations such as a flat, low tone, or V-shaped curve with unusually good discrimination for speech considering the loss is sensorineural (see Glossary, Chapter 19);
4. A sensorineural loss that begins insidiously in early or middle adult life and progresses relentlessly with no known cause;
5. On otological examination a pinkish blush, or red dis-coloration of the promontory, seen through the intact and normal eardrum of one or both ears (Schwartze's sign).

None of these are very strong points on which to base a diag-nosis and the determination of a fixed stapes, whilst it can be inferred from the stapedial reflex test, can only be positively diagnosed at surgery.

The recent development of high resolution computerised tomographic scanning has allowed evaluation of the state of the bony labyrinth in patients with presumed cochlear otosclerosis, and it appears that areas of bony resorption around the cochlear and vestibular labyrinth can be easily seen in these cases but not in controls. This method will therefore probably become a confirmatory diagnostic investigation in the near future (de Groot, Huizing, Damsma, Zonnereld and Van Waes 1985).

As with syphilis, the diagnosis of otosclerosis causing vertigo or unsteadiness is not just academic as prolonged use of sodium fluoride does seem to improve the vestibular symptoms. The rationale for using fluoride is that it appears to slow down resorption of bone when used in large doses (Bretlau, Causse, Causse, Hansen, Johnsen and Salomon 1985). In clinical trials, which in the main have been retrospective and often uncon-trolled, 40 to 60 mg of sodium fluoride have been given per day for periods of at least 6 months with remission of vestibular symptoms in the majority of patients. However, otosclerosis is a disease whose passage is measured in decades rather than in years and the long-term results may not be so favourable. Nevertheless, in a condition for which there is no other treatment, a 6 month trial of sodium fluoride could well be worth-while.

PAGET'S DISEASE

Paget's disease is a chronic, progressive non-fatal disease of the skeleton occurring in the later years of life with no known cause. It is not uncommon, and is characterised by active bone resorption and irregular deposition of new bone occurring at the same time. There is increased fibrosis leading to a hypertrophied vascular demineralised bone. This is rather like the pattern seen in otosclerosis but Paget's is a widespread disorder and the serum alkaline phosphatase becomes raised in the course of the disease, whereas otosclerosis is focal and limited to the temporal bone.

The vestibular and cochlear portions of the labyrinth can be involved to produce a collection of symptoms just like Ménière's disease, with a sensorineural deafness, tinnitus and episodic vertigo. There may well be a conductive element in the hearing loss due to involvement of the bony walls of the middle ear and the ossicles, when cochlear otosclerosis with vestibular symptoms might be considered as a diagnosis. In those patients with skeletal deformity and bone pains the diagnosis is obvious — sometimes the bony changes are limited to the skull and temporal bone and the patient will be otherwise asymptomatic. The diagnosis then becomes more difficult unless you remember Paget's disease, when a plain skull x-ray and the serum alkaline phosphatase are diagnostic. The first change on the skull x-ray is a sharply circumscribed zone of bone resorption but later on the greatly thickened fluffy appearance of the skull bones is typical.

The progression of the hearing loss is slow (about 2.0 dB per annum on the average of the threshold at 500, 1000 and 2000 Hz when compared to age matched controls — about 0.5 dB per annum) (Baraka 1984). The caloric responses appear to be normal, even in those with a Ménière's-like syndrome (Morrison 1975).

Treatment is difficult. It had been hoped that the introduction of calcitonin would alter the progression of the laby-rinthine Paget's but controlled studies show this not to be the case at least as far as the hearing is concerned (Walker,

Evanson, Canty and Gill 1979). Nevertheless, if the patient is disabled by the vertigo and other disease, especially syphilis, has been excluded, then a trial of calcitonin over a period of months could be considered.

DRUG-INDUCED DIZZINESS

Anyone who has organised a drug-trial with a placebo group included will know that dizziness is one of the commonest reported side-effects of the inert compound. Little wonder then that some text books of ENT practice contain sections extending over many pages which list drugs that may cause dizziness. These lists seem to encompass almost every drug you would ever want to prescribe and are really of little value. Nevertheless, contained within them are groups of drugs that really do cause problems and it is these that will be discussed here. Drugs that cause central effects and neuropathies leading to unsteadiness will be discussed in later chapters.

Drugs damaging the labyrinth

The introduction of streptomycin into clinical use in 1945 soon resulted in a flurry of reports of disturbance of balance and a description of the vertigo induced by the drug even finds its way into a novel (Ellis 1958). Since then, all of the aminoglycosides have been found to have some effect which is either predominantly vestibular or cochlear (Table 11.1). The reasons for this selectivity are unknown. The damaging effects of the aminoglycosides are accentuated if there is renal failure as the drug is only excreted in the urine and blood levels therefore rise. The drugs themselves are toxic to the kidneys so will further enhance renal failure resulting in even higher levels unless carefully monitored. The aminoglycosides are in the whole available as intramuscular preparations and so tend to be used in hospitals, and most people are aware of the potential problems although cases of vestibular damage still occur when it has been necessary to use the drug in life-threatening infections. Following recovery from the illness the vestibular failure is noted and is usually symmetrical and progressive so that the symptoms of oscillopsia may occur with the surroundings apparently moving

145

Table 11.1: Relative toxicity of the aminoglycosides

	Vestibular	Cochlear
Streptomycin	++++	+
Dihydrostreptomycin	+	++
Netilmicin	?+	?(+)
Sisomicin	?++	?+
Gentamicin	+(+)	+
Amikacin	+	++
Kanamycin	+	+++
Tobramycin	+	++++
Neomycin	+	+++++

up and down on walking (see Chapter 2). Gross unsteadiness can also arise with the patient having to walk carefully in the light but being completely unable to maintain balance in the dark or with his eyes closed. The condition is untreatable. During treatment vertigo can occasionally occur if the labyrinths fail rapidly and the symptoms cannot be distinguished from vestibular neuronitis, although sustained nystagmus is not usually present since the condition is bilateral. There is often, however, a jerky horizontal movement of the eyes during the acute phase with an inability to hold lateral gaze positions that may mimic nystagmus although if observed carefully the slow drift and rapid flick are absent.

Other ways of poisoning people with the aminoglycosides have also been developed. The drug is absorbed in large quantities through burnt skin and open ulcers and the use of various sprays and lotions which contain aminoglycosides have frequently resulted in permanent deafness and occasionally vestibular failure (Table 11.2). This is especially relevant in extensive burns where there is often an element of renal failure. To be fair to the manufacturers, the labels on the tins or on the product information slips do contain the information, but unfortunately the effect of the drug may be delayed in onset and progressive so that by the time deafness or vertigo are developing it is already too late to stop treatment.

Although aminoglycosides are not absorbed through healthy gut after oral administration, their use to sterilise the bowel in liver failure (to reduce the risk of hepatic encephalopathy) or inflammatory bowel disease has led to a number of cases of deafness and vertigo.

Table 11.2: Commonly used topical preparations containing an aminoglycoside

	Proprietary name	Aminoglycoside
Ear and Nose Drops:		
	Framycort/Framygen	F
	Sofradex/Soframycin	F
	Cidomycin	G
	Garamycin	G
	Genticin	G
	Gentisone HC	G
	Betnesol N	N
	Neo-Cortef	N
	Predsol N	N
	Vista Methasone N	N
	Audicort	N
	Otosporin	N
	Triadcortyl	N
Topical skin preparations whose proprietary names are not listed above:		
	Sofratulle	F
	Betnovate N	N
	Gregoderm	N
	Hydroderm	N
	Dermovate NN	N
	Stiedex LPN	N
	Neomedrone	N
	Adcortyl with Graneodin	N
	Silderm	N
	Cicatrin	N
	Graneodin	N
	Myciguent	N
	Polybactrin	N
	Tribiotic	N
	Nybadex	N

Abbreviations: F, framycetin; G, gentamicin; N, neomycin.

The introduction of the powerful loop acting diuretics (etha-crynic acid, frusemide and bumetanide) brought a new and completely unsuspected hazard. These drugs occasionally caused deafness, tinnitus and vertigo, especially when given intravenously and when there was concurrent renal failure. This was tolerable since the symptoms were usually transient but the completely unexpected twist was that there was a remarkable synergy between the loop diuretics and aminoglycosides in caus-ing profound damage to the inner ear when the dosage of either was thought to be quite safe. It is likely that renal damage also occurs. The mechanism of the interaction is still unknown but the drug manufacturers wisely state on most of the instruction sheets that the loop diuretics and aminoglycosides should not be given together. Nevertheless, this combination is frequently used in intensive care units and the vestibular troubles that occasionally occur are unfortunate and probably avoidable side-effects as, nowadays, the newer penicillins and cephalosporins have a wide-enough range and bactericidal action to cope with most problems.

As a general principle, it would seem sensible to avoid the use of the aminoglycosides unless absolutely necessary especially when there is raw skin, disordered guts or renal failure, and to try very hard never to give loop diuretics at the same time.

12

Disorders of the Neck and Dizziness

The neck contains a whole range of structures which can all conceivably cause dizziness if damaged or deformed. The cervical spine consists of seven cervical vertebra, each of which has a number of facets for articulation with the vertebrae above and below or in the case of the uppermost 1st cervical vertebra (the atlas) for articulation with the skull above. Not only does the spinal cord pass through the vertebral canal but the verte-bral arteries, one on each side of the neck, also traverse separate foramina in the transverse process of each vertebra. The right and left vertebral arteries arises from their respective subclavian artery and enter the foramen of the 6th cervical vertebra. Each ascends almost vertically through the spine accompanied in its course by sympathetic nerve fibres and a meshwork of small veins. When it leaves the atlas it turns sharply backwards then winds around the lateral mass of this the first vertebra to enter the skull through the foramen magnum. It then runs up the front of the brainstem for a short distance before meeting the other vertebral artery to fuse and form the single basilar artery. This continues on for a short while before splitting into the two postero-cerebral arteries which form part of the circle of Willis (Figure 12.1).

Inside the skull the vertebral and basilar arteries have several branches which supply the brainstem, cerebellum and occipital lobes of the cerebrum. The branches are inconstant as to their origin from vertebral or basilar, may occasionally be absent and some are end arteries supplying areas with no collateral circu-lation. The names are not really important to us but the struc-tures that they supply are, for dizziness is a frequent companion of disorders of these vessels.

Figure 12.1: Schematic view of the vertebro-basilar system and its branches. The vertebral arteries run through bony canals in the cervical spine and are prey to a number of conditions such as atheroma or cervical spondylosis that can drastically reduce the size of the vessel lumen. The branches of the vertebro-basilar system are named and from the posterior cerebral artery two communicating branches go to form the circle of Willis.

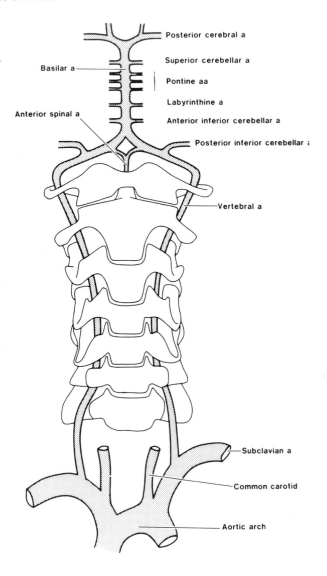

(Table 12.1 shows the distribution of the branches of the vertebro-basilar system to parts of the brain that are important in normal balance.)

The neck and cervical spine also contain many muscles and joints with their associated somatosensors and the sympathetic chain in addition to the arteries supplying important parts of the brain. All of these structures have at some time been implicated as a cause of dizziness.

How real these suggestions are is a difficult problem. Certainly, involvement of the vertebral arteries by atheroma may cause transient ischaemia of the brainstem when the neck is turned or extended. The patient complains that symptoms arise during a manoeuvre such as watching an aeroplane pass overhead, stretching up to hang out the washing, or even downing the last drops from a pint beer-glass. The most commonly presenting feature is vertigo, that is usually rotary and short-lived, but alterations of vision with a greying or cloudiness also occur and sometimes the sensation of a luminous appearance before the eyes with a zig-zag, wall-like outline — the so-called fortification figures, or teischopsia — may arise. Occasionally the patient collapses, often to be thought drunk by those around him if he has been finishing a drink.

Whether consciousness has been momentarily lost is often difficult to decide, but some patients do and some do not, although fortunately there seems to be nothing more serious involved in those who do. The vertigo is usually so scary that the

Table 12.1: Arterial branches of the vertebro-basilar system

Posterior inferior cerebellar:	Cerebellum
	Lateral part of medulla
	    incl. vestibular and cochlear nuclei,
	    spino-cerebellar tract

Medullary:	Medulla
Pontine:	Pons
Labyrinthine:	Inner ear
Anterior inferior cerebellar:	Cerebellum
Superior cerebellar:	Cerebellum

Posterior cerebral:	Occipital pole and infr. temporal
	    region
	    incl. visual areas of cerebral
	        cortex

151

individual has to take things quietly, even lie in bed for the rest of the day. Many other symptoms can make an appearance during the episode although surprisingly transient deafness is rarely ever mentioned. Double vision, headache, weakness, a slight slurring of speech all can be present for a short while, but these and other symptoms fade so that between attacks the patient is quite normal and clinical examination is unrewarding. It is sometimes possible to induce nystagmus with certain neck positions and this can be recorded by electronystagmography, thereby confirming the clinical suspicion. X-rays of the cervical spine looking for osteophytes or disc protrusion are not of much value since there is such a range of deformity in the asymptomatic population.

Provided there is a good history of symptoms relating specifically to neck movement, then little else needs be done other than suggesting avoidance of the provoking situation or perhaps even the prescription of a stiff collar for a short while to train the individual not to make extreme movements. However, should the attacks be spontaneous, then it is more likely that episodes of transient ischaemia of the brainstem are occurring and these need further work up and referral as they may just be the forerunner to a full-blown brainstem infarct. These conditions will be discussed in Chapter 14 on brainstem disease.

As to the other structures in the neck that might cause dizziness, the evidence is less certain. There is no convincing work that can implicate the sympathetic chain at least in man, whilst there are results suggesting that the various receptors in muscles and joints may play some role at least in experimental animals. Destruction of the posterior roots of the upper cervical nerves, i.e. the sensory roots, can cause disorders of balance and produce spontaneous and positional nystagmus (Biemond and de Jong 1969). In addition, once the nystagmus and imbalance that results from a unilateral labyrinthectomy has settled when compensation is complete, subsequent destruction of the cervical input results in a return of the original features. In man, anaesthetising the muscles and joints of the neck with local infiltration of an anaesthetic results in the sensation of being pulled to the side of the infiltration, a tendency to lean to that side, and when lying flat a feeling of tilting also to the same side (de Jong, de Jong, Cohen and Jongkees 1977). Whether the same conditions apply in cervical osteoarthritis, or following injuries to the neck is difficult to decide. Whiplash injuries to the neck are very commonly incriminated as a cause of persisting vertigo and unsteadiness following injury. We have already seen in Chapter 6 how this sort of trauma can result in small bleeds and patchy oedema in the brainstem which are cause enough for the symptoms. There are, in addition, abnormalities in caloric function in the great majority of patients who sustain this sort of indirect head trauma, something that did not occur in the experiments when local anaesthesia was injected into the joints and muscles of the neck. Overall, the evidence for a direct involvement of the neck in the persisting post-traumatic vertigo and dizziness of whiplash injuries is scanty although derangements of sensory input from the neck may play some part in the delay in recovery. A good stiff collar may be needed to help the neck pain that arises from trauma, and as a side-effect reduce vertigo and unsteadiness.

In general, a reasonable way out of the dilemma as to whether the neck is to blame or not would be to place the diagnosis of 'cervical vertigo' at the bottom of your list of possible diagnoses and to exclude labyrinthine damage or disease first. An abnormal caloric response would mean that the seat of the trouble is probably the ear or the brainstem and that changes in the neck receptors are contributing to the feeling of dizziness. This means that in spite of reservations about cervical vertigo there are a group of people who are helped by wearing a collar and if so, a short trial may be worthwhile.

13

Growths in the Cerebello-Pontine Angle

Between the temporal bone and the brainstem lies the cerebello-pontine angle (CPA), a small elongated almost slit-like space filled with cerebrospinal fluid. Across the CPA runs a cluster of cranial nerves on their way to the internal auditory meatus in the temporal bone. These are the cochlear and vestibular divisions of the VIIIth cranial nerve and along with them the facial (VII) nerve. At the top of the CPA is the trigeminal (V) nerve and its semilunar (or Gasserian) ganglion. At the base are IX, X and XIth nerves passing out of the skull through the jugular foramen. Running along the floor is the abducent (VI) nerve at the start of its long journey to the lateral rectus muscle of the eye. The inner wall and roof of this region comprise the brainstem and parts of the cerebellum respectively. Thus within a small space are several important neural structures, and to make matters worse, a complex network of blood vessels — the vertebral and basilar arteries and their branches.

Tumours growing in this region are not particularly common and form less than ten per cent of all primary intracranial tumours. There are, however, some important features that distinguish this region from the rest of the inside of the skull. Whereas the order of frequency of primary intracranial tumours is, in general, gliomas (commonest), meningiomas, then neuromas, in the CPA the order is reversed with some additional oddities making an appearance. This is important because neuromas are benign tumours, although their situation close to the vital centres in the brainstem makes them potentially and sometimes actually, very dangerous as of course can be the surgical removal. Nevertheless advances in surgical and anaesthetic techniques have made safe removal of even the larger neuromas feasible, although the earlier the surgery the less the risk.

I will start with a description of the commonest of the 'neuromas' that grows in this region and trace the symptoms and signs that arise as its size increases and eventually comes to press upon the brainstem and cerebellum and to cause raised intracranial pressure.

ACOUSTIC 'NEUROMAS'

Acoustic 'neuromas' have the distinction of being doubly misnamed. First they are nearly always found on the vestibular nerve and second they are not neuromas as such but tumours of the nerve sheath and should properly be called neurilemmomas. However the name acoustic neuroma is entrenched in the literature and will be used here. A small subgroup of acoustic neuromas is found in association with von Recklinghausen's disease which is a familial neurofibromatosis. As well as the café-au-lait patches on the skin, neurofibromata are found on peripheral, spinal and cranial nerves. Individuals thus afflicted are prone to develop acoustic neurofibromata which are frequently bilateral. In addition, meningiomas, angiomas and tumours of the cell layer lining the hollow central canal of the spinal cord and brain — the ependymomas — can also arise in von Recklinghausen's.

The early growth of an acoustic neuroma occurs in the portion of the nerve that lies in the bony internal auditory meatus (IAM). As the size increases the structures within the canal become compressed and this brings on the early symptoms. A progressive unilateral deafness is most common and it is often associated with tinnitus. Occasionally tinnitus in one ear only may be the first symptom. The deafness may increase so gradually over one or two years that the symptoms are ignored or accepted. Frequently there is a sense of discomfort or a very slight ache about the ear on the involved side and this may also be relegated to 'catarrh' or some other indistinct cause. Although the tumours are growing on the vestibular nerve vertigo is uncommon since compensation occurs for the slow loss of function. Bouts of unsteadiness on sudden head movement or fleeting episodes of short-lived vertigo may be present early on in the course of the growth but tend to settle as time passes. The prolonged repeated attacks of vertigo as found in

Ménière's disease are not a feature of acoustic neuromas. However, the arterial supply to the inner ear runs through the IAM and, having provided an adequate blood flow despite external compression, can suddenly fail due to a small increase in pressure from the tumour. The result is a sudden deafness, possibly a crashing tinnitus and a bout of profound vertigo or unsteadiness that lasts for several days. The deafness and tinnitus may improve a little but the suddenness and severity of onset of the vertigo usually forces the patient to seek attention.

Surprisingly the facial nerve is barely affected by small tumours and its motor fibres are resistant even to extensive stretching when large tumours are present. The sensory and secretomotor fibres are more sensitive and the occasional patient will notice an alteration in taste, sometimes a dry eye and even less frequently an overproduction of tears and a wet eye.

At this stage with the tumour lying within the meatus or just protruding a little into the CPA diagnosis may be difficult. The patient has a sensorineural hearing loss that can be demonstrated by whisper and tuning fork tests, and confirmed by pure tone audiogram. Unfortunately the pattern of this loss — high tone, low tone or flat — is unhelpful, and there are no simple audiometric tests that are diagnostic of the condition.

In small tumours spontaneous nystagmus is sometimes present but is usually suppressed by optic fixation. It is a very fine horizontal nystagmus, with the fast phase to the opposite side on looking to that side, that is its first degree. Using Frenzel's glasses or the ophthalmoscope removes the optic fixation and sometimes allows the nystagmus to be seen. More helpful is a simple cool caloric test where the great majority of patients have a greatly reduced or absent response to irrigation on the deaf side. A bi-thermal caloric defines the problem more precisely and a severe canal paresis with or without a directional preponderance is found. The ability to produce tears as shown by a Schirmer's test can either be reduced or enhanced on the deaf side and it might just be possible to detect loss or impairment of taste by simple means.

At this stage the other cranial nerves are normal on testing but the combination of neural deafness and a poor response to caloric testing should warrant referral for a specialist opinion. Despite various sophisticated audiometric test regimens, the diagnosis of tumours of the internal auditory meatus and CPA can only be made by radiology. A reasonable plan would be to perform linear or polytomography first as this clearly shows the bony walls of the internal meatus. These walls are frequently expanded by the growth and it is this change that can usually be detected (Figure 13.1).

The advent of computerised tomography (CT) has made the diagnosis of these tumours easier and in some centres a posterior cranial fossa CT scan with intravenous enhancement is the first radiological investigation. Not only can this show bony changes but in the case of a larger tumour will often show expansion of the growth into the CPA. When clinical suspicion of small tumours is high the CT scan can be combined with an air meatogram whereby a small quantity of air is introduced into the spinal canal via a lumbar puncture. Cerebrospinal fluid is removed at the same time and sent for estimation of its protein levels which are frequently raised when acoustic neuromas are present. The patient is then tilted so that the air ascends to the CPA and the CT scan repeated. With skilful technique air fills the CPA and penetrates the internal auditory meatus outlining the nerves. If a tumour is present this fails to occur and its outline is shown instead (Figure 13.2).

The relative ease with which small tumours can be identified has of course brought with it problems of management. Should all small tumours be removed as soon as they are diagnosed? At this stage the patient is relatively symptom-free and despite major improvements in technique, surgery is not without hazard. The risk of a facial nerve palsy may be too great for the patient to accept when not much seems to be wrong.

As time passes, the tumour expands into the CPA and other symptoms arise in addition to the deafness and tinnitus. The trigeminal (V) nerve can be involved and the patient may just notice slight changes in the perception of light touch and temperature when washing their face or applying make-up. Tinglings or numbness are common but frank pain is rare although the onset of trigeminal neuralgia is sometimes reported. In this condition the pain, which usually involves the face rather than the forehead, comes on as a series of short, sharp but intense stabs, each stab lasting a few seconds or minutes. These attacks cluster together over a few hours and then are replaced by a pain-free interval. A new attack occurs and the pattern repeats itself. When acoustic neuromas or other CPA tumours are the cause of this irritation to the nerve the

Figure 13.1:
(a) Plain x-ray tomograms of the internal auditory meati (IAM).
The arrows indicate the upper and lower limits of the canals on
each side and on the right side they are marginally wider. A
small acoustic neuroma was present.

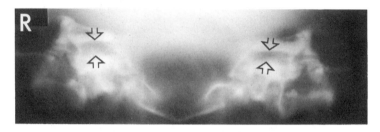

(b) Here, there is gross widening of the right IAM again indicated
by the arrows. This was caused by a large acoustic neuroma.

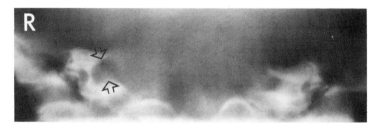

(c) A computerised tomographic scan, at right angles to the
'cuts' in the plain tomograms, showing widening this time of the
left internal meatus.

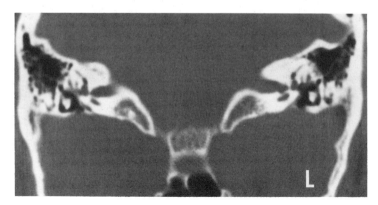

Figure 13.2: (By courtesy of Dr P. Phelps, radiologist at the Royal National Throat, Nose and Ear Hospital.)

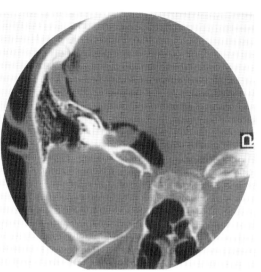

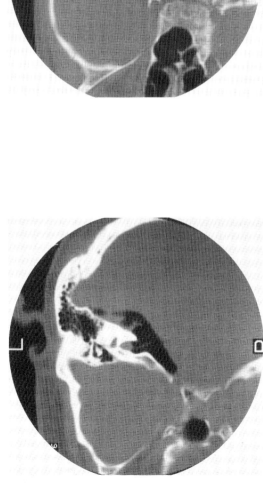

(a) An air meatogram showing the posterior cranial fossa and internal auditory meatus of the left ear. Air — which shows up black — has entered the internal meatus, outlining the nerves and revealing a small tumour at the apex of the canal. (b) A much larger acoustic neuroma has been outlined by the air and can be seen filling the internal meatus and extending into the posterior fossa.

Figure 13.2: (c) This is a magnetic resonance scan with Gadolinium enhancement and reveals the same small acoustic neuroma that was shown by the air meatogram. Magnetic resonancing with enhancement is non-invasive, does not involve the use of x-ray and may in future be the investigation of choice.

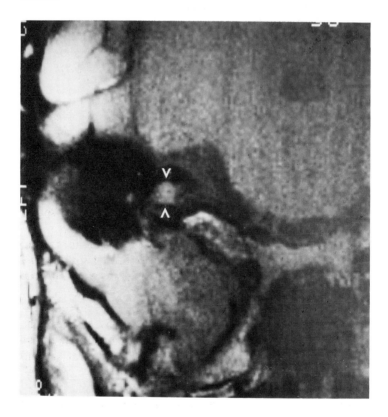

attacks may be persistent and resistant to treatment unlike the idiopathic variety where remissions and response to carbamazepine are almost the rule. During the attacks the sufferer will often screw up one side of the face as the pain arrives and reaches its brief climax. This involuntary contortion gives the condition its alternative name of tic douloureux.

The detection of Vth nerve sensory loss is probably best seen in the early stages by the loss of the corneal reflex, an easily performed and sensitive test.

The loss of other cranial nerves, VI, IX, X, XI, comes much

later in the course of the disease and by this time symptoms and signs of brainstem or cerebellar compression are usually apparent.

A dull occipital headache, the exact cause of which is uncertain, is common, as is the onset of increasing unsteadiness. There may have been slight unsteadiness provoked by unusual movement during the early phases of the disease but now the patient is becoming persistently troubled, and has difficulty walking properly and in straight lines. Occasionally clumsiness of one leg makes its appearance. 'My foot doesn't know what to do.'

Examination at this time will reveal the deafness, absent caloric function on the same side, probably a loss of the corneal reflexes but, in addition, there will usually be some spontaneous and abnormal eye movements. The most common pattern at this stage is a fine vestibular type nystagmus with the fast phase to the good ear when looking in that direction, that is, a first degree nystagmus. This is found in combination with a much coarser and slower nystagmus, variable in amplitude and speed, towards the involved side. This coarse nystagmus is thought to be due to direct cerebellar involvement. As the brainstem and other vestibular pathways become compressed all sorts of disordered eye movement can make an appearance so that the diagnosis of central involvement becomes much easier.

Other cerebellar signs may be detected. Tests of co-ordination in the hand and arm sometimes reveal ataxia, but when the legs are tested with the patient lying on a couch and running the heel of one foot along the shin of the other leg from knee to ankle and back again then the result is clearly abnormal. Straight line walking may be quite impossible.

By now further compression and distortion of the brainstem is occurring and transient episodes of double vision occur as the abducent (VI) nerve is stretched. These episodes can give way to permanent effects as the lateral rectal muscle fails to function adequately, although the slight palsy needed to produce the diplopia may not be visible on examination.

Raised intracranial pressure

Hopefully patients with acoustic neuromas or other CPA tumours will have presented themselves to a doctor before the complications of raised intracranial pressure (RICP) arise. The early literature on acoustic neuromas is full of descriptions of end-stage disease, and even nowadays there appear to be two groups of patients who differ not in the disease but in the stage at which they present. The late presenters end up at the neuro-surgeons whilst the early ones are seen by an ENT surgeon. This probably accounts for the differences in the descriptions that can be found in the literature with the neurosurgeons' patients barely seeming to resemble those of their ENT counterparts.

Nevertheless a description of the features of RICP is in place here as it forms such an important part of many other conditions, and by itself can cause vertigo and unsteadiness. Any expanding space occupying lesion inside the skull will eventually cause RICP, so that the symptoms and signs that occur can be separated into those specific to the site of involvement, and those caused by the generalised effects of RICP. I have described the specific features that arise from tumours in the internal auditory meatus and CPA, but these could easily be replaced by those typical of involvement of any other part of the brain: the features of RICP would be more or less the same wherever the causative growth.

Cerebrospinal fluid (CSF) is relentlessly produced within the ventricles of the brain to pass out through several foramina and flow around the brainstem, cerebellum and cerebral hemispheres. It probably also passes down the spinal canal to a limited extent. Obstruction to the free passage of CSF by the sheer size of the tumour in the CPA eventually results in a rise of CSF pressure with secondary effects on the brain.

The localised discomfort around the ear changes into a diffuse, dull, aching pain that increases in intensity as the days pass by. Next to come are nausea and vomiting that usually first make their appearance in the mornings, but increase in severity so that they can last most of the day. These two symptoms arise from irritation of the emetic centres in the brainstem and do not need to appear together. Effortless vomiting without, or preceding the nausea is not uncommon. Together these two symptoms can usually be settled by various centrally acting anti-emetics such as the phenothiazines, and there is a risk of obliterating warning symptoms by inappropriate treatment, especially if a proper examination has not been performed.

As grey matter becomes compressed, 'awareness' decreases and the level of consciousness declines. This can be a vague area with imprecise words such as drowsy, stupor, semi-coma, and so on, being used in an attempt to define how alive or dead the patient is. Various schemes have been devised to quantify this level and often one hospital will use a chart designed in-house for this purpose. The Glasgow Coma Scale (Teasdale and Jennet 1974) defines the coma level on the basis of three responses. First, the ability of the patient to open their eyes spontaneously, in response to speech (not necessarily the command 'open your eyes'), to pain or not at all. Second, the best verbal response ranging from orientated through confused, inappropriate words, incomprehensible sounds to none. Third, the best motor response the top of the scale being obeys commands, the bottom being no response with localisation, flexion, then extension to pain lying in between. There are many modifications of this format, each with their own particular advantages and disadvantages.

Accompanying this change in consciousness and probably affected by it is a decline in the intellect. There is poor thinking, loss of recent memory, bad judgement and shortened attention span.

Vertigo, unsteadiness and double vision if not already caused by a CPA tumour will almost certainly appear as intracranial pressure increases and the brainstem is squeezed.

After the intracranial pressure has been elevated for some days or weeks oedema of the optic nerve occurs and this can be seen with the ophthalmoscope as papilloedema. The first change is filling up of the region in the middle of the optic disc from which the vessels emerge. The disc then becomes pinkish and loses the distinct margin at its medial edge and then all around. The vessels are distorted as they bend round the enlarged optic disc and the veins are engorged. Subsequently optic atrophy occurs with the disks becoming pale and white yet still having an indistinct margin.

The changes are all described in relative terms and if you have not bothered to observe at least some normal optic fundi in the past it might be difficult to make the diagnosis with confidence.

With persisting papilloedema, vision not unsurprisingly deteriorates, but this is nearly always preceded by repeated, fleeting loss or dimness of vision — an unhealthy symptom given the sonorous name amaurosis fugax. With some tumours outside the CPA, raised intracranial pressure may be the major

163

feature as the growth is in a relatively silent area of the brain. The combination of headache, vomiting and papilloedema is ominous and implores urgent referral to a neurosurgeon.

As death approaches, further signs of brainstem distortion occur. The occulomotor (III) nerve is involved and one or both pupils dilate, and fail to respond to light. A persistent fever and alterations in pulse rate and blood pressure develop. These last changes also appear during a rapid rise in pressure that occurs after an intracranial bleed — perhaps an extradural haematoma following a head injury. And for this reason alone you should remember that the pulse falls and the blood pressure rises (the opposite to that which occurs in profound blood loss elsewhere).

The other practical point to remember concerns monitoring the neurological progress of someone who is unconscious because of a head injury. It is of no use asking the nursing staff to record the pupil reactions, pulse and blood pressure if you do not tell them to call the doctor when certain changes occur. The offices of medical insurance companies are probably littered with charts showing the pulse rate dropping below the rising systolic blood pressure to form the so-called 'cross of death' after which recovery is unlikely.

OTHER CPA TUMOURS

Other tumours can occasionally arise in the CPA, and may be difficult to distinguish from accoustic neuromas on history alone. Neuromas on the Vth nerve typically produce facial symptoms before deafness but this is unreliable. Meningiomas may produce more headache and more trigeminal neuralgia but are usually identical at presentation to typical moderate-sized acoustics.

However with both of these growths the caloric function is usually intact and the x-ray changes are helpful. Meningiomas typically have calcification within and around them and this is often seen on plain films and nearly always on CT scans. Widening of the foramen ovale and erosion of the apex of the petrous bone suggest a Vth nerve neuroma.

CPA cholesteatoma is not the acquired sort described in Chapter 5 but a congenital type that probably arises from islands of squamous epithelium in or around the temporal bone misplaced during the genesis of the inner ear. It is rare but can mimic the acoustic neuroma, with vertigo or unsteadiness as one of the presenting features. These cholesteatomas have a typical appearance on CT scans with a scalloped edge and a very low density.

14

The Brainstem

As far as we are concerned, there are three major conditions or groups of conditions that can involve the brainstem to cause dizziness. These are:

1. Disorders of the blood supply;
2. Disseminated sclerosis;
3. Metastatic deposits from malignant tumours.

The effect that drugs can have, both directly and indirectly, is discussed in Chapter 17.

DISORDERS OF THE BLOOD SUPPLY

The disorders that affect the blood supply range from vertebro-basilar ischaemia (resulting from kinking of the vertebral arteries during extension of the neck and already described in Chapter 12) through migraine to transient ischaemic attacks and a completed stroke. The vessels supplying the brainstem also supply the cerebellum and nearby cerebrum so that depending on the extent of the involvement by the disease a wide constellation of symptoms and signs can arise.

Migraine

Migraine is a common condition affecting perhaps one in twenty of the population and seemingly involving females more than males. The age of onset is between five and thirty years in the vast majority of sufferers and two-thirds have a family history of a similar disorder. The cause is quite unknown, although virtually every conceivable condition affecting mankind has at some time been incriminated. However, there do seem to be certain foods and drugs that set off an attack, and hormonal changes related to the contraceptive pill, periods or the menopause, flickering lights or loud noise are also well-established provoking agents, although psychological factors are probably the most common and possibly most potent. An inability to achieve at home or at work what is demanded by the patient's personality, especially if there is a hint of real or imagined unfairness, results in frustration which has a very good chance of invoking an attack.

The features of migraine arise from an instability of the small arteries that supply the brain, meninges and scalp. The outcome is a disturbance both of the brain itself, which gives rise to the aura, and of the pain-sensitive coverings that result in the headache.

The classic form of migraine comprises an aura followed by the headache, and there is usually little problem in recognising the condition from this pattern. In other people the headache occurs alone or the aura may have occurred only two or three times in the course of many years. The reverse with an aura being the major feature is less common and can cause confusion if the headache is minor and ignored, or absent.

The most common features during the aura are visual with either a distortion of normal sight consisting of shimmering, double vision, perhaps a patchy loss of the visual field or the addition of abnormal features such as moving spots or lights, zig-zag outlines around luminous centres, displays of colours and so on. Often the two are mixed. Other sensory disturbances are common with numbness and tingling of the face, lips, hands or feet. Sometimes one-half of the body may be involved. Disorders of thinking, speaking, reading and comprehension are also seen. Abdominal disturbances with feelings of discomfort, fullness, emptiness even colic are reported. Tinnitus and a feeling of fullness in the ear may arise. Rarely major motor symptoms and a fleeting paralysis of one-half of the body or of one limb may make an appearance. Permanent major neurological damage is however very rare.

The aura usually lasts for some minutes and then the headache develops. This is a dull throbbing pain that is unilateral in two-thirds of patients. It is made worse by movement, rather like the headache of a severe hangover, and spreads out gradually across the head. It can start at the front or back of the head and once established usually lasts the rest of the day. Nausea and vomiting, more often than not, accompany the beginning of the headache whilst a profound diuresis and a feeling of well-being, out of character for the sufferer, may individually or together be present as the headache fades.

Not surprisingly, vertigo and unsteadiness may develop during a migraine attack, as the blood supply to the brainstem is compromised. The symptoms can arise during the aura, during the headache, which is probably the commonest presentation, or even in the headache-free periods, although other pathology may be at work coincidentally to the migraine. For vertigo to arise as the headache departs is rare.

A form of migraine arising from involvement of the brainstem blood supply has been described by Bickerstaff as 'Basilar Artery Migraine' (Bickerstaff 1961). It is found predominantly in adolescent girls and usually occurs around the time of their periods. The aura lasts from a few minutes to three-quarters of an hour and consists of vertigo, unsteadiness (which may occur by itelf), slurred speech, tinnitus, tingling around the lips and hands and visual disturbances, usually manifest as flashing lights or loss of vision. As the aura fades an occipital headache develops, usually with nausea and sometimes with vomiting which seems to lessen the intensity of the headache. This collection of symptoms is fairly clear-cut and, as with the vertigo that arises during the aura of a classic migraine, when auditory symptoms can also be present, the diagnosis is not a problem.

Usually the vertigo and unsteadiness arise during the course of the headache and may even persist for as long as the headache, thereby confining the patient to bed. It appears that during the migraine attacks that are triggered by periods or the menopause, vertigo and unsteadines are amongst the commonest and most severe symptoms, and are often the reason for visiting the doctor rather than the headaches which are tolerable or simply treated.

Another group comprises those with migraine who develop bouts of vertigo without headache, between their typical attacks. These bouts may be accompanied by other symptoms of an aura, especially tinnitus and hearing loss, when it might be impossible to distinguish the condition from Ménière's disease.

The vertigo can be transitory or last several hours and, if associated with periods, may persist for up to a day or two. These attacks have been called migraine equivalents and are presumably failure of a migraine to develop fully. In some, the history of earlier completed attacks helps in the diagnosis but in others where there are no past migrainous features the diagnosis is presumptive and should only be made after other conditions have been excluded.

Even though the history may be typical of migraine, a thorough neurological examination is a must for two reasons. First, to exclude any gross neurological defects, since between attacks the owner of the migraine is normal. Many workers, however, found that those with severe vertigo are likely to have some defects when sophisticated vestibular testing is carried out. Presumably the alterations in the blood supply that occur during attacks result in small changes to the very sensitive structures of the labyrinth or to the vestibular pathways in the brainstem that are detectable but are adequately compensated for between attacks. The second reason for a complete examination is for reassurance. To be suddenly struck by flashing lights, vertigo and a pounding headache conjures up the worse fears even in the most phlegmatic of individuals, and to be shown and told that there is nothing life threatening going on often helps overcome their fears.

Occasionally, however, some other condition causing the symptoms is present with aneurysms, angiomas, and malformations of the intracranial blood supply being favourites. The early stages of rising intracranial pressure, from a whole list of causes, can also produce migraine-like symptoms, but in all these conditions there is often an unusual presentation of the migraine, or perhaps a neurological sign that will warrant referral for a specialist opinion. The onset of an occipital headache, vertigo and vomiting for the first time may be the result of a subarachnoid haemorrhage and suspicion of this should also lead to referral for investigation. Finally, as we will see in the next section, transient ischaemic attacks involving the brainstem can produce symptoms similar to those of a migraine and the differentiation, if the onset is later in life, may be impossible. Assessment of risk factors for stroke — obesity, smoking, diabetes, hypertension — should therefore be carefully evaluated and corrected if possible.

Having excluded other causes of the symptoms, you can now

embark on management, confident in your diagnosis. Reassurance is essential in the first instance and may need to be reinforced from time to time by another complete neurological examination, if the attacks cannot be well controlled. The history may have revealed precipitating factors and some, like foodstuffs and oral contraceptives, can be withdrawn. This is especially important as far as 'the pill' is concerned, as it seems to increase the, albeit slight, risk of permanent neurological damage in migraine sufferers. Reserpine, viloxazine and dipyridamole occasionally precipitate attacks and should be replaced (Nightingale 1985). If the migraine is incapacitating, a change in lifestyle might just help, and some find relief from alternative medical treatments.

Since the cause of migraine is unknown, no specific therapy is available but the nausea and vertigo often respond to vestibular sedatives, which may need to be given other than orally if there is vomiting. During the early stages of the aura, rebreathing from a paper bag may just prevent the full-blown attack as the raised carbon dioxide levels overcome the intracranial vasoconstriction. Simple analgesics are often effective enough for the headache especially if given with metaclopromide to speed up gastric emptying and subsequent absorption.

If the attacks are frequent enough then various prophylactic drugs can be tried, and many may have to be prescribed before one is found that is effective for the individual (Table 14.1).

Transient ischaemic attacks

As you will have realised from the preceding section and from that on vertebro-basilar insufficiency, the symptoms and signs

Table 14.1: Prophylaxis of migraine

None of these drugs are effective during an attack	
Propranolol:	40 mg b.d. or t.d.s., may need 80 mg or more. Other betablockers can be tried.
Clonidine:	0.5 mg mane increasing slowly to 0.5 mg t.d.s. Can be taken in one dose at night time. May cause drowsiness.
Methysergide:	Only if severe migraine that cannot be otherwise controlled. 1–2 mg t.d.s. for maximum of 6 months then at least one month off medication. Peripheral vasoconstriction, retroperitoneal, pleural and cardiac fibrosis can occur.

that arise from reduction of the blood flow to the brainstem and the nearby cerebellum and cerebrum are fairly consistent and it is the pattern of their presentation and associated features that help sort out the underlying disease. Transient localised failure of the blood supply occurs when short-lived 'soluble' platelet thrombi are launched into the general circulation from atheromatous plaques, and land up in the small arteries that branch from the vertebro-basilar system. They lodge here long enough to cause symptoms before dissolving or breaking up and passing on. In the brainstem the nuclei and neural tracts are tightly packed and the blood supply is not always clearly lateralised so that odd concoctions of patchy symptoms and signs may arise.

The patient, who is usually a man past middle age frequently has other signs of arterial disease with angina or claudication being common as are co-existing hypertension and diabetes. Careful enquiry usually fails to uncover a precipitating factor that can be ascribed to each incident which may even come on at rest. The symptoms last for minutes or hours before fading and vertigo is the commonest complaint. It can take almost any form and is associated with a feeling of unsteadiness, difficulty in walking and, if severe enough, with vomiting. Next in frequency come visual disturbances with blurring, double vision and partial loss of the visual fields. There is often an associated headache so that the picture described sounds like that of an 'old man's migraine'. Many of the other symptoms of migraine can also arise with uni- or bilateral tingling of face, arms or legs, occasionally a weakness of the limbs, slurred speech, difficulty swallowing and tinnitus being amongst them. Involvement of the vessels that supply structures near the midline can result in drop attacks in which postural tone is lost and a fall to the ground occurs without loss of consciousness. Control is regained rapidly and the individual is able to get up again, shaken and stirred but usually without damage.

The attacks can happen many times a day or only infrequently. Others have clusters of attacks over a few hours or days before occlusion becomes complete and a formal stroke develops. The major importance of transient ischaemic attacks is that they signal the existence of significant cerebrovascular disease and indicate the potential danger of cerebral infarction, although this risk is not so great when the brainstem, rather than other portions of the brain are involved.

171

During the attacks, neurological signs relating to the presenting symptoms can be found, and some may even persist between attacks. The most common signs are a spontaneous nystagmus that can be typical of peripheral or central vestibular involvement, or be a confusing mix of both; disorders of movement of the palate and tongue, a paralysis of some of the extraocular muscles and a peripheral sensory loss and weakness.

The ophthalmoscope should be used to look for changes in the retinal blood vessels. The pulses may be absent or unequal in the legs, suggesting atheroma, as does the presence of systolic bruits over the carotid arteries in the neck and xanthomata in the skin. Check the blood pressure and take blood for blood sugar estimation. You may also want to determine whether the patient has hyperlipidaemia as this, together with cigarette smoking and hypertension, is certainly a powerful risk factor for coronary artery disease if not for cerebrovascular problems. The measurement of hyperlipidaemia is unfortunately not quite straightforward. The patient must be fasting, in otherwise normal health and not on a strict weight-reducing diet. He must also not have had a heart attack within the three months before the sample is taken which must be performed without venous stasis. The request form should ask for at least the serum cholesterol and triglycerides (see Slack 1983).

The firm diagnosis of transient brainstem ischaemia is of course impossible as there are none of the identifying features that occur with other conditions and no definitive tests. Nevertheless, on the presumption that the clinical picture fits, the patient must be warned of the risks of smoking with his condition and told to stop. He must be encouraged and helped to lose weight if obese and have his hypertension and diabetes treated, where appropriate. Lipid lowering drugs should not be used until all the above features are well under control, and vestibular sedatives are not first-line treatment although they may be useful as an additional measure in prolonged bouts of dizziness.

Completed strokes

Cerebral infarction resulting from occlusion by emboli or thrombosis around atheroma cannot be distinguished by the neurological disorders they produce although embolic episodes tend to occur suddenly whilst thrombotic ones often have a stuttering progressive onset typically over a few hours. Bleeds into the brainstem from aneurysms, vascular malformations and hypertensive vascular disease arc less common but, in general, are much more serious and frequently progress rapidly from headache to unconsciousness and death. They will not be considered further.

The exact picture that arises from infarction depends on the area that has been damaged. Since the arterial supply to the brainstem is highly variable and the degree of overlap between different branches varies from person to person, a range of combinations of symptoms and signs can arise. This has given rise to many named syndromes which, although bestowing immortality on the originator does little for our understanding. More recently, there has been a tendency to dispense with the names and concentrate on the neurological patterns that occur and relate them to the normal anatomy. As far as vertigo is concerned, the regions involved are the lateral portions of the brainstem and the associated features depend on how far up or down this structure the infarction occurs.

The most commonly presenting pattern involves the medulla, and the patient complains of vertigo, headache, nausea, vomiting and hiccoughing. There is usually blurred vision (sympathetic), difficulty speaking (IX, X) and difficulty swallowing (IX, X). There is frequently a Horner's syndrome (sympathetic) with drooping of the eyelid, a small pupil, retraction of the eyeball, and loss of sweating on the same side of the face. Classically loss of pain and temperature sensation over the same side of the face (V) and opposite upper half of the body are described but apparently are not so often noticed by the patient (Rudge 1983).

The examination will show that the patient is unsteady on his feet and has a tendency to veer off to the same side as the lesion when he tries to walk. The neurological defects are usually obvious on testing and there is a horizontal nystagmus with the fast phase to the opposite side. Bithermal caloric testing does not show a canal paresis but does reveal a marked directional preponderance. Whilst deafness can occur in infarction further up the brainstem in the pons when the cochlear nuclei or even the labyrinth itself are involved, it does not occur in lateral medullary involvement. Lateral pontine damage frequently involves the VII nerve so that a facial palsy results whilst sparing IX and X.

As time passes, the symptoms of laterally medullary infarction may gradually improve and many of the neurological defects resolve. With lateral pontine infarction the patient may remain vertiginous as not only have the vestibular nuclei been involved but so also has the labyrinth, and compensation may not occur especially in the elderly. Rudge (1983) reports that persisting benign paroxysmal positional vertigo and nystagmus can also be present, presumably because of the labyrinthine damage.

Once established, no routine medical treatment has been shown to improve recovery from a stroke which either does or does not occur by itself. Anticoagulation to present further thrombosis requires that you should know that a bleed is not the cause of the trouble. You will only be certain in patients with established mitral valve disease and atrial fibrillation when the likelihood of an embolus is very high. For the rest dropping the blood pressure in the overtly hypertensive is probably best delayed until at least three weeks after the initial incident to avoid further spread of the infarct through poor perfusion. The management of the patient who deteriorates, having stabilised after the initial problem, is more difficult and referral to a neurologist or neurosurgeon may be in the patient's best interests. For the majority of patients the only role the doctor can play is to organise supporting services so that recovery can occur without complications (Langton-Hewer and Wade 1984). In brainstem infarction there is commonly aspiration of food because of motor and sensory disturbances in the pharynx and larynx. A liquid diet should be avoided and semi-solid foods that can be chewed and formed into a bolus that is easier to swallow be advised. A temporary naso-gastric tube might be needed to overcome the initial problems with swallowing.

The subclavian steal syndrome

Although not very commonly encountered, the subclavian steal syndrome is at least amenable to treatment and is said to occur in about 3 per cent of patients with symptoms of vertebro-basilar insufficiency. The root of the trouble is stenosis or occlusion of the first part of the subclavian artery before the origin of the vertebral artery (Figure 14.1). If there is partial occlusion then at least some blood flows along the subclavian artery and

Figure 14.1: Schematic view of the carotid artery system showing the typical sites of stenosis. In the subclavian steal syndrome a stenosis is present at the origin of the left subclavian artery. Use of the left arm brings about an increased requirement for blood and this is thought to be met by a shunting of blood from the left vertebral artery.

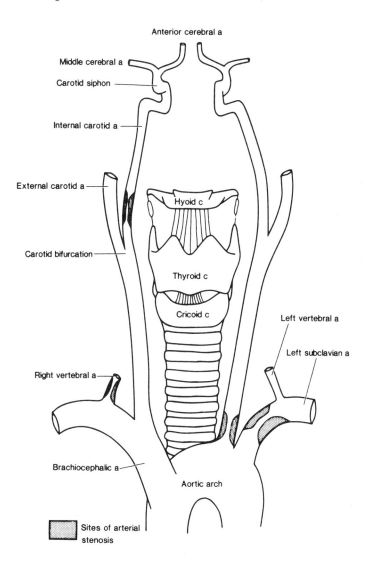

at rest is sufficient to supply the arm. During strenuous exercise involving the arms — on the same side as the stenosis — flow is inadequate through the stenosis and blood is siphoned from the vertebral artery which now becomes the major source of supply to the arm on the involved side. The subclavian therefore steals blood from the vertebro-basilar system and this causes poor perfusion of the brainstem, cerebellum and parts of the cerebrum. With complete occlusion, all the blood supply to the arm is derived by way of the vertebral which drains the opposite vertebral and probably the basilar as well.

The history associated with subclavian stenosis is fairly typical and the condition affects men and women in their middle 50s and onwards about equally. Aching and weakness occur in the arm of the involved side during exercise which can also bring on a bout of vertigo. Sometimes the symptoms are precipitated by turning the neck. Associated with the vertigo can be all or a few of the other symptoms of brainstem ischaemia. Visual problems can arise with blurring, double vision and partial transitory loss being common, although visual hallucinations are not. Headache, weakness, clumsiness and dysarthria can all accompany the dizziness which may be terminated by a 'drop attack'.

Physical examination between attacks usually reveals a weak or absent radial pulse on the involved side and there is usually a difference in the systolic pressures of more than 30 mm Hg between the two arms. When the occlusion is partial, a bruit may be detectable above or over the clavicle.

The stenosis can be detected by arteriography and if the patient's symptoms are severe and their general health good enough then endarterectomy and reconstruction are nowadays reliable procedures.

DISSEMINATED SCLEROSIS

Most nerve fibres are surrounded by a sheath of myelin, interrupted at regular intervals by short myelin-free stretches or the nodes of Ranvier. The myelin sheath endows the insulated nerve with a more rapid conduction time and the nodes act to enhance the travelling electrical signal by further depolarisation in the form of an action potential. Myelin is a complex collection of lipids and lipid-protein complexes and is unfortunately prone to destruction in a number of conditions that together form the demyelinating diseases. These are a mixed bunch ranging from the demyelination that can follow immunisation and bacterial or viral infections to the most common form — disseminated sclerosis (DS) and its variants. Unfortunately there are no specific diagnostic tests for DS and since the condition can present in many ways it is difficult to define precisely. Nevertheless the symptoms and signs generally reflect involvement of central myelin with lesions separated in time and space. No specific causal agent has been found, and although many aggravating factors have been suggested — pregnancy, surgery, trauma, emotion, infections and immunisations — none have been implicated beyond doubt.

The disease commonly presents in young people without any other systemic disorder as a series of neurological events spread over a variable time interval and which cannot be explained on the basis of any other single pathology. Central 'white matter' is usually involved with supranuclear weakness, inco-ordination, paraesthesiae and visual complaints being common. Signs of involvement of 'grey matter' — aphasia, seizures, fasciculation and atrophy — are much rarer, but the psyche may be involved in one-third of patients.

The disease is usually chronic with exacerbations and remissions occurring over a number of years and it is this pattern of disease that is most likely to present with some form of dizziness. Other patterns can be fulminating with a rapid decline to death over a few weeks or a chronic form that unremittingly progresses over a few years. Overall the symptoms depend on which part of the central nervous system is involved in the demyelination process and as a first symptom dizziness is common (Table 14.2).

Table 14.2: Occurrence of first symptoms in DS — often occurring in combination

	Percentage
Weakness	50
Diplopia, impaired vision	20
Tremor, ataxia, inco-ordination	20
Paraesthesiae	30
Vertigo	10
Sphincter disturbances	5

A single severe prolonged attack of rotary vertigo made worse by movement, rather like that which occurs in vestibular neuronitis can occur, but frequent, less severe bouts are more common. Either pattern occurring as a presenting feature or early in the course of the disease can cause confusion with other conditions especially if there is disease in the ears.

The severe attacks last for many days or weeks before improvement begins. The nausea settles and the effects of head movement diminishes. Cochlear symptoms are rarely mixed with vestibular ones and are surprisingly uncommon by themselves. Presumably this occurs as the auditory pathway diverges widely after the cochlear nerves reach their nuclei in the brainstem so that the lesions of DS cause few symptoms although they may be detectable with sophisticated tests of auditory function.

The vertigo may however, be accompanied by other symptoms especially tingling or numbness in one or all of the limbs. Weakness is common but if generalised may not be considered as unusual after a week-long spell of vertigo and vomiting. A dropped foot, a weak hand, even a complete paralysis of one arm or leg takes you closer to a tentative diagnosis. The combination of vertigo with the rapid onset of a painful loss of vision in one eye makes the diagnosis almost certain, since retrobulbar neuritis is hardly ever caused by any condition other than DS.

So in taking the history ask about episodes of tingling, weakness, clumsiness, difficulty with passing water or incontinence. All these are valuable positive clues, whilst headache or transient difficulty with speaking are rarely part of the pattern of DS.

Although vertigo must be the most distressing form of dizziness that arises in DS other types occur more often. Double vision coming on quickly brings with it marked unsteadiness as does blindness, weakness or loss of sensation in the legs.

Examining the patient with vertigo during the acute phase often reveals spontaneous nystagmus that can be horizontal and direction changing, or vertical — the latter two confirming its central origin. When the vertigo has settled and the nystagmus is abating a positional nystagmus can sometimes be induced on testing and is found to reduce, stop or even reverse the residual spontaneous nystagmus. Later on, if the spontaneous nystagmus stops, a central type of positional nystagmus may be found. Continuing nystagmus without vertigo or even without a history of its occurrence is sometimes noticed indicating the compensation has occurred for the damage that demyelination has caused within the vestibular pathway.

As far as the other physical signs go there may be impairment of vibration sense and joint position sense in the legs or even the arms, while skin response to touch and pin-prick are spared. If there is weakness, then there are usually upper motor neurone signs with spasticity and rigidity, exaggerated tendon reflexes and upgoing plantars.

The failure of co-ordination causes poor performance in tests of fine movement and the finger–nose procedure reveal a marked tremor on trying to touch the examiner's finger tip with their own — the so-called intention tremor. Walking may also be affected with stiff-legged, wide-based unsteady movements — the spastic-ataxic gait. The ataxia can also involve eye movements so that while attempting side to side movements the eyes come to reach their final position in a series of jerky stepwise movements that often overshoot the intended position. (This has been called ataxic nystagmus but as mentioned in Chapter 4 this term contradicts itself.)

Another fault of eye movement that occurs in DS, and is most commonly caused by DS, is an inter-nuclear ophthalmoplegia. Demyelination in the median longitudinal fasciculus results in a relative loss of ability to move either eye across the midline towards the nose. There is therefore inability fully to adduct either eye, or if nystagmus is also present then it is diminished or even absent in the adducting eye compared to the other abducting eye.

The caloric tests are nearly always abnormal if vertigo has been present, but if there is spontaneous nystagmus they may be difficult to interpret. However when this settles or if allowances are made then there is usually some combination of a canal paresis and directional preponderance or one or other alone.

The occurrence of vertigo or unsteadiness during the course of strongly suspected or diagnosed DS causes little problem in additional diagnosis if the ears are healthy. As a single presenting feature without other neurological or general symptoms or signs it may be necessary to give the label 'vertigo of unknown origin' and see the patient at intervals to check for other developments to give substance to a final diagnosis.

Meanwhile, during the acute vertigo any of the range of vestibular sedatives and anti-emetics may need to be tried. Some authorities feel that a short course of steroids in high dosage may help in reducing the severity of the acute problem whilst acknowledging that they have no real place in the long-term management of the condition.

METASTATIC DEPOSITS FROM MALIGNANT TUMOURS

Primary tumours in the brainstem are rare and deposits from distant growths occur much more frequently. They make their appearance either as a late manifestation of a widespread carcinomatosis — when diagnosis is relatively easy — or as the first warning of an unrecognised malignancy elsewhere. This primary site can be almost anywhere but lung and breast are common as are gut, genito-urinary tract, bone and thyroid.

Any tumour growing inside the skull produces its effects by a combination of the specific symptoms and signs that arise from the site of the lesion itself and later on when the mass is bigger or is obstructing the passage of CSF problems arise as the intracranial pressure is increasing. The features of raised intra-cranial pressure have been described in the preceding chapter and vertigo and unsteadiness are amongst them. The specific effects caused by brainstem deposits can be varied and bizarre but an almost invariable hallmark is their persistence. Compen-sation usually always occurs in labyrinthine change but if the pathways that mediate compensation are involved then the signs if not the symptoms persist.

Progressive unsteadiness or the onset of an unpleasant vertigo will frequently bring the patient to the doctor. The vertigo which is made worse by movement persists for days or more usually weeks before slowly settling. The physical signs however linger on.

Spontaneous nystagmus can be horizontal, vertical or rotary and is inhibited by eye closure or darkness. The direction of the nystagmus may change as the eyes are deviated first to one side then the other. There are frequently associated disorders of eye movement with squints and sometimes an internuclear ophthal-moplegia making an appearance. Positional nystagmus of a 'central type' can be found sometimes with quite alarming nystagmus in a patient who is untroubled by the procedure. Occasionally the positional nystagmus is the only physical sign although on caloric testing a canal paresis or directional prepon-derance are common.

So far the pattern of the vestibular upset described in this section has not differed a lot from that described for DS. It is the accompanying features that may help you make the distinction, and mean that you need to take a full history and perform a thorough general examination. Even then you might be no wiser and so should send sputum for microscopy for malignant cells, urine for analysis for blood and casts and faeces for the detection of occult blood. Follow any leads with the appropriate radiological or endoscopic examination and sometimes a cause will show itself. Frequently nothing is to be found and then time and follow-up makes the answer clear.

Although primary tumours of the brainstem are rare in adults they are some of the more common childhood tumours along with those in the cerebellum. Nearly all are glial tumours with medulloblastomas being the most common. A progressive unsteadiness, perhaps the development of a squint should alert you to look closely for spontaneous nystagmus, which is frequently present, and have the child referred quickly for a neurological opinion and CT scanning.

15

The Cerebellum

The cerebellum occupies the bulk of the posterior cranial fossa and sits on the brainstem to which it is attached by a superior middle and inferior peduncle on each side. The gross anatomical separation of the cerebellum into two lateral and one median lobe (the vermis) does not reflect its physiological division into one group of structures dealing with equilibrium and another dealing with the regulation and co-ordination of movement. Failure of the latter portion — the neocerebellum — gives rise to many detectable abnormalities. Some of these have been described in Chapters 2, 3 and 4, and so are only mentioned by name here. The other features are described more fully.

1. Hypotonia shows itself by flaccidity of muscles, lessened resistance to passive movements and floppiness. Some of these features can be shown by having the patient stand, eyes closed, with arms outstretched palms down in front of them. The back of one hand is then given a light downwards tap. In the normal the hand will bounce back after a short excursion but with cerebellar disease, and on the side of the lesion, the arm will drop considerably and be unlikely to return to its starting point.

2. Abnormal posture. The shoulder often droops on the affected side; the trunk may be bent a little to the same side and rotated to the good side so that the drooping shoulder is a little forward of the good one. Sometimes the head is rotated and flexed. If the disease is severe posture cannot be maintained and the patient tends to fall to the side of the lesion.

3. Ataxia takes several different forms:

a. Dysmetria: where the range of movement is inappropriate for the action intended, so that finger overshoots the target when the patient is performing a finger–nose test;

b. Tremor on voluntary movement: so that fine precise movements are difficult to perform;

c. Dysdiadochokinesis: which is the inability to perform alternating movements rapidly and precisely;

d. Rebound: if a normal person is asked to flex his elbow against resistance and then this resistance is suddenly released, the forearm travels only a short way as the triceps contracts. In cerebellar disease this reaction is sluggish or absent and the hand swings up to hit the patient's shoulder, or, if the positioning is wrong, the patient's face;

e. Abnormal reflexes: the loss of adequate co-ordination results in characteristic changes seen when the tendon reflexes are tested. These are best demonstrated by the knee-jerk performed with the patient sitting on the edge of the couch with his calves and feet hanging in the air. Tapping the patellar tendon on the affected side gives the expected response but this is followed by several pendulum-like swings of the leg;

f. Nystagmus;

g. Disordered speech;

h. Abnormal gait: have all been described earlier.

Disease in those parts of the cerebellum that are involved with equilibrium — the paleocerebellum and flocculo-nodular lobe — causes swaying, staggering and stumbling. Not surprisingly, vertigo can also develop during acute problems and not be, subjectively, any different from that which arises from disease in the labyrinth or brainstem.

Unfortunately for the patient many of the symptoms of cerebellar damage do not express themselves when the cause is a slowly progressive lesion such as a tumour. This presumably occurs because there are compensatory pathways available that become active whilst cerebellar function is being lost. Although this might delay diagnosis in those with insidious disease it is a blessing for those with acute problems since significant functional recovery can occur.

Many rare and peculiar conditions can involve the cerebellum and this book is not the place to describe them since, if dizziness occurs at all, it is only a small part of the presentation. However, other more common problems do arise and children with cerebellar disease may be taken to the doctor with the parents complaining that the child is dizzy because he or she staggers and falls.

THE SPINOCEREBELLAR DEGENERATIONS

The spinocerebellar degenerations are a group of closely related disorders that are usually familial, but which may also occur sporadically. They present as progressive disorders of gait, posture, balance and movement. The pathology is a degeneration of the long ascending or descending tracts in the spinal cord or of the cerebellum and cerebellar peduncles. In some syndromes, both spinal and cerebellar pathways are involved. Occasionally degeneration occurs in other parts of the central nervous system so that a remarkable collection of symptoms and signs can arise. This has allowed many physicians to attain posterity by having their name attached to the first description of one particular combination of features. The aetiology of the degenerative process is unknown.

The spinal forms of the disease often present in childhood with stumbling and awkwardness. This is not unlike the unsteadiness that can occur in glue ear where both middle ears are full of thick viscid mucus. However, the unsteadiness progresses, there are sometimes associated skeletal deformities, and as the degeneration advances the child's walking becomes markedly ataxic, whilst later on the trunk is involved so that the body itself sways irregularly from side to side and from front to back when movement is attempted. The arms and speech are finally involved in the ataxic process.

Most forms of childhood spinal degeneration are familial although the occasional sporadic case turns up in adolescence or early adult life when it has to be distinguished from disseminated sclerosis presenting as weakness in both legs. Although there is no specific treatment for either the prognosis is generally better for those with DS. Differentiation is usually made from the progressive nature of the condition and the loss of tendon reflexes which is nearly universal in the spinal degenerative diseases.

The cerebellar degenerations usually appear later in life and have a 'core' of cerebellar symptoms and signs. There is ataxia of the trunk legs and arms, dysmetria, action tremor, dysdiadochokinesis, and sometimes a static tremor.

Many of these are familial and progress relentlessly with no specific treatment available. However, there are some cases that have a different origin although the pathology seems to be the same.

Alcoholism is the commonest alternative cause and there is a subacute onset of unsteadiness developing over a few weeks or months. The patient walks slowly and lurches around, and the heel–shin test reveals gross ataxia in the legs. However, there is little or no involvement of the arms and nystagmus and dysarthria are usually absent. Having reached this stage the condition appears to stabilise although other features of central or peripheral alcoholic poisoning may make their appearance. The diagnosis and management of alcoholism are described more fully in Chapter 16.

A similar but more extensive cerebellar degeneration can be one of the non-metastatic effects of carcinomas arising usually in the lung or ovary (Brain and Wilkinson 1965). The patient complains of rapidly increasing unsteadiness, but in addition the arms soon become clumsy and speech deteriorates as dysarthria and dysphonia develop. One of the many varieties of cerebellar nystagmus develops in about half the sufferers. The cerebellar symptoms often precede those that arise from the primary site and so specific examination is important in patients who are unsteady and ataxic but who have no signs of sensory loss. A chest x-ray is necessary and if this is clear and you do not feel competent to palpate an ovarian mass then the patient should be referred for a gynaecological opinion.

The organic mercurial compounds are commonly used to combat fungal disease of cereal crops, and as additives to paints to prevent the growth of mould. By accident they can find their way in excessive amounts into the body. The non-organic mercurial compounds can similarly be assimilated as they are still fairly extensively used in certain paint colours like vermilion and as an anti-fouling agent for ship and boat paints. Toxic levels of mercury regularly cause cerebellar degeneration so that unsteadiness and tremors are common. In addition excessive salivation and a metallic taste in the mouth arise and the teeth become loose. A bluish discoloration is found at the edges of the gums. The psyche also alters with the individual becoming shy, withdrawn and irritable — hence the term 'mad as a hatter' since mercuric salts used to be used in felt-making. The kidneys can also be involved with proteinuria and sometimes a complete nephrotic syndrome developing. The diagnosis is usually straightforward on the history and examination but is confirmed by finding urinary mercury levels to be more than 0.1 mg per litre. Normal values are up to 0.001 mg per litre. Treatment is very important to stop further progress of the renal disease, and requires removal of the source of mercury in the first instance. Penicillamine may be helpful in enhancing urinary excretion but the use of other chelating agents has not been found to be helpful.

Recovery is slow even after removal of mercury from the body and the persisting cerebellar ataxia may make a return to normal living impossible.

POST-INFECTIVE CEREBELLAR DISEASE

Following viral infections, especially in infancy, an encephalitis involving the cerebellum occasionally makes its appearance. A generalised viral upper respiratory tract infection instead of settling progresses to profound unsteadiness with ataxia and a staggering, stumbling gait. Some or all of the other signs of cerebellar disease develop and finally after some weeks or months resolve with a variable degree of residual loss. The condition has been dignified with the title 'acute cerebellar ataxia of infancy' and is usually associated with an influenzal illness although the coxsackie and echo viruses may be involved in a similar condition that presents in adults. Measles sometimes causes the condition, whilst chickenpox does so only rarely.

CEREBELLAR HAEMORRHAGE

The cerebellum is supplied by the posterior inferior, anterior inferior and superior cerebellar arteries. Bleeding from any one of these results in cerebellar infarction. For a few days preceding the catastrophe there may have been some minor warning symptoms of occipital headaches, short-lived vertigo or clumsiness before the full-blown syndrome develops. There is profound vertigo, ataxia, vomiting and a severe occipital head-ache. Some of the sufferers will sooner or later lose conscious-ness.

On examination, there is often a coarse nystagmus and some-times a peculiar 'ocular bobbing' where the eyes rapidly deviate downwards then slowly drift back to the central position. However, there are few specific signs localising the bleed to the cerebellum and none indicating brainstem involvement. The caloric responses are usually intact.

This combination should suggest the diagnosis which warrants urgent referral to a neurosurgical centre for CT scan-ning and evacuation of an intracerebellar haematoma. Unlike bleeds into many other parts of the brain, surgical exploration and removal of the haematoma will often save life and reduce morbidity. Do not be tempted to perform a lumbar puncture to make a diagnosis unless you have neurosurgical assistance standing by, for the risk of cerebellar herniation and rapid death is high.

CEREBELLAR TUMOURS

Tumours pressing on the cerebellum from the outside have been described in Chapter 13, and this section deals with tumours growing from within.

With primary and secondary cerebellar tumours, specific cerebellar symptoms are often minimal or absent until the growth is far advanced. This is particularly unfortunate since the cerebellum is a common site for tumours, especially in child-hood. Medulloblastomas occur in the first decade of life, astro-cytomas in late childhood and early adult life, whereas haeman-gioblastomas are nearly always found in the cerebellum and are associated on rare occasions with an angioma of the retina and cystic lesions in the pancreas and kidneys when the condition is termed von Hippel-Lindau disease.

Medulloblastomas are initially midline tumours but the other types can be midline or lateral as can secondary deposits. The symptoms that develop depend on the location of the tumour within the cerebellum but with all tumours symptoms of raised intracranial pressure are common presenting features. Head-ache, vomiting and nausea are the cardinal complaints whilst papilloedema is usually obvious on observation.

187

Midline tumours

The cerebellar signs with midline tumours are specific effects on walking and standing because of truncal ataxia. The child lurches from side to side with feet spaced widely apart. Unsteadiness and vertigo are mixed together and, on testing, the child falls backwards or forwards. There are few signs of ataxia or weakness in the arms or legs when tested with the patient sitting or lying, and nystagmus is often absent. If these signs are present in addition, then there is involvement of the lateral parts of the cerebellum. If the child is young, the raised pressure may have caused enlargement of the skull with separation of the suture lines.

Lateral tumours

Like the midline tumours, those laterally placed may present with raised intracranial pressure but there is in addition: failure of co-ordination in the limbs on the affected side, nystagmus, headache and an abnormal posture. The patient is unsteady and clumsy and tends to topple over to one side. The limbs on that side are floppy on testing and all of the signs of ataxia (dysmetria, intention tremor, dysdiadochokinesis and rebound) can be present. Nystagmus is common but surprisingly speech is hardly ever disordered in either midline or lateral tumours. A dull occipital headache extends down to the top of the neck and the patient may stand in the abnormal shoulder drooped posture described earlier in this chapter. Vertigo on turning the head is commonly present.

Cerebellar tumours are those brain tumours most amenable to surgical removal since most, if not all, of the cerebellum can be removed without disabling post-operative morbidity. Indeed, in children the brain seems to compensate so well that eventually compensation may allow them to lead a normal life.

16

Peripheral Neuropathies

This chapter could be filled with well-remembered, but rarely seen, syndromes that have an annoying tendency to crop up at clinical examinations since the physical signs, known to the examiners, may be difficult for the students to detect. Instead I will describe the more common conditions that sometimes cause a loss or reduction of sensation and power in the legs and which may result in unsteadiness. Like most neurological works a list of causes is included in Table 16.1. Whilst far from complete this list tries to emphasise those causes of peripheral neuropathy that can present with unsteadiness and which can often be diagnosed by simple means. Many of the conditions are found in the elderly whose vestibular systems are not quite as efficient as

Table 16.1: Peripheral neuropathies likely to result in unsteadiness

Causative factors:
Alcohol
Diabetes
Chronic uraemia
Drugs: Isoniazid
      Nitrofurantoin
      Vincristine
      Gold
      Allopurinol
Organic chemicals and solvents
Heavy metals — arsenic
Vitamin deficiencies: B complex
              B_{12}
Non-metastatic effects of carcinoma
Hypothyroidism
Spinal cord — stretching, compression or disease

those in the young, so that the addition of a peripheral neuro-pathy can render the individual quite unsteady and house-bound. Some of the conditions can be treated with an improve-ment in the neuropathy and a reversal of the unsteadiness. So, before you accept or claim that it is the patient's age that is causing the trouble, try to eliminate at least the relevant condi-tions described below. If a sensory neuropathy in the legs cannot be reversed then simple aids such as a pair of walking sticks to enhance somatosensory input by way of the arms, the avoidance of thick, soft-soled shoes and the prescription of effective spectacles to optimise sight can all help to reduce the disability.

ALCOHOLIC PERIPHERAL NEUROPATHY

There is no clear agreement as to the features that need to be present for a diagnosis of alcoholism to be made. This problem is neatly demonstrated by the various attempts that have been made to define an alcoholic. These range from that of the heavy drinker with problems who claims that an alcoholic is 'someone who drinks more than I do' to that of the World Health Organi-sation which describes alcoholics as:

Those excessive drinkers whose dependence upon alcohol has attained such a degree that it shows a noticeable mental disturbance, or an interference with their bodily and mental health, their interpersonal relations and their smooth social functioning; or those who show prodromal signs of such development.

Whatever definition you care to use there is no doubting the enormity of the problem with an estimated 300,000 alcoholics in England and Wales, and alcoholism being the commonest cause of a peripheral neuropathy in Western medical practice. Alcohol directly poisons nerves but the secondary nutritional deficiency effects are probably more important. Vitamin B_1 (thiamine) deficiency is almost certainly the major culprit, but a generalised insufficiency of the rest of the B vitamins and a deficiency of dietary proteins play some part.

The loss that comes with alcoholism is mixed but is mainly sensory, at least in the early stages, when the patient complains of numbness, tingling and odd unpleasant creeping sensations, in the feet especially, in the calves sometimes and occasionally in the hands. Pain is typical and can be severe with burning and cramp-like sensation in the calves, which is especially severe at night. Sometimes the pain is absent. It is the loss of sensation that gives the feeling of walking on cotton wool with consequent unsteadiness, especially in the dark. If the alcohol intake continues, weakness makes a more obvious appearance and the unsteadiness progresses to an inability to climb stairs or even to walk at all.

The generalised examination may reveal some of the other signs of alcoholism, although many manage to stay in good shape. Obesity, flabbiness, dilation of the small blood vessels around the nose and eyes, a coarse tremor of the outstreched hand and a large liver are all pointers to the condition.

In the legs the skin is red, shiny and dry, but the feet are often very sweaty, a feature that may make its presence obvious even before the shoes are removed. Pain on pressing the calves is nearly always present as is the absence of ankle tendon reflexes. The patellar reflexes may be difficult to detect even with the patient enhancing the response by pushing his hands together hard as the reflex is tested. All forms of sensation are symmetrically reduced in the feet, calves and thighs, the upward extent varying from person to person.

Ataxia as shown by the heel-shin test is present, not as a result of cerebellar disease, but because proprioception and maybe power, are abnormal. The Romberg's test is positive with increased unsteadiness as the eyes are closed.

Simple blood investigations can be helpful. Signs of liver involvement are shown by an elevated level of plasma gamma-glutamyl transpeptidase (syn. tranferase). This level returns to normal fairly quickly after a period of abstinence and so may not be helpful. However a macrocytosis of the red cells, in the absence of any anaemia, is a consistent finding and this is shown as a raised mean cellular volume (MCV) of more than 93 femto litre (fl). The exact level depends on local laboratory standards and calibration. Since the turnover of red cells is slower than the recovery time of the liver during abstinence the macrocytosis persists for one or two months and is a good marker of the condition (Wu, Chanarin and Levi 1974).

None of these signs are specific to an alcoholic peripheral neuropathy, and perhaps now is the time to delve more deeply into the rest of the patient's life to establish the diagnosis, for alcoholism is a series complaint. Alcoholics tend to have more social, psychological and physical disabilities than the rest of the world.

Social problems

Heavy drinking frequently causes marital problems with a wife complaining that her husband tends to be stupidly embarrassing at parties, that he is boastful, sulky, given to tall stories and is a flirt. This can eventually grind down a relationship and exert a strong influence on the children (Orford 1977). Work can also suffer as alcoholics are absent more often and are dismissed more frequently than their non-alcoholic colleagues. Surveys of individuals involved in accidents, both domestic and on the road have usually shown high blood alcohol levels in a significant percentage. Drunkenness also seems to be related to crime, and although a criminal record does not mean alcoholism, excessive drinking prior to imprisonment is remarkably common.

Psychological problems

The depression that is directly due to alcohol may be increased by the social failure and poor health that frequently attend the habit, and this results in an increased rate of actual and attempted suicide. Deterioration of the personality, intellectual impairment, black-outs after heavy drinking bouts and short-term amnesia are all common. Hallucinations may occur without the other symptoms of delirium tremens, which typically starts soon after withdrawal of alcohol, begins at night and lasts for two or three days. Fear, restlessness and illusions and hallucination may all be present and there is an associated tremor and ataxia. A raised pulse and blood pressure and a fever accompany the symptoms.

Physical disability

Many systems can be affected by alcohol. Damage to the liver and gastrointestinal tract produces indigestion, heartburn, vomiting, diarrhoea, bleeding and jaundice. The heart and lungs suffer with palpitations, chest pains, bronchitis and pneumonia being common. Hormonal and metabolic changes result in obesity with striae, breast hypertrophy in men, reduced libido (in spite of outward expression of the opposite) and infertility.

Any of these features presented in isolation or as a small cluster may mimic other diseases and initiate expensive and fruitless investigations. Assembling all the background inform-ation helps to complete the jig-saw that indicates a heavy alcohol intake. During the course of questioning, perhaps when you are asking about medications or smoking habits, the daily or weekly amount of alcohol consumed should also be sought. If heavy drinking is suspected and the answers are evasive do not ask 'are you an alcoholic' because although the very occasional individual will break down in relief at being found out, you will alienate the vast majority. Perhaps you should aim ridiculously high if they are unhelpful and suggest, say, two bottles of spirits a day and then reduce to the level at which agreement is made.

The CAGE questions (Mayfield, McLeod and Hall 1974) are often helpful:

1. Have you ever felt that you should cut down on your drink-ing?
2. Have people annoyed you by criticising your drinking?
3. Have you ever felt bad or guilty about your drinking?
4. Have you ever had a drink first thing in the morning to steady your nerves or get rid of a hangover?

with two out of four positive replies identifying a good propor-tion of problem drinkers.

The patient is unlikely to 'come clean' and tell all, unless he admits the problem to himself and feels secure in talking to the doctor. The management of alcoholism is beyond the scope of this book but the British Medical Journal book *Alcohol Prob-lems* (1982) is very useful and worthwhile reading. An alcoholic neuropathy can recover completely, although slowly if absti-nence is maintained. Hospital admission, withdrawal of alcohol, control of the DTs if they arise, and treatment with multivitamin preparations including thiamine (B_1), riboflavine (B_2), nicotin-amide and pyridoxine (B_6) should be the starting point if permanent sensory and, worse, motor loss is to be avoided.

DIABETIC NEUROPATHY

Diabetics can suffer from a variety of neuropathies. The less common forms include a mono-neuritis multiplex where in association with atherosclerosis and small vessel disease, isolated often painful lesions of peripheral nerves occur. Sciatica, wrist drop (ulnar nerve) and double vision (III, IV, VI cranial nerves) are typical. A separate autonomic neuropathy can cause disturbances of gut motility, a dry shiny tight skin and postural hypotension.

A peripheral neuropathy is probably present to a certain degree in most diabetics. It may be asymptomatic and only detectable on testing of nerve conduction velocities, or show itself as a symmetric mainly sensory neuropathy involving the legs. Burning or shooting pains may be present, especially at night and the soles of the feet are often very sensitive so that walking is unpleasant. Vibration and joint position sense are impaired or absent at the feet, ankle, shins and sometimes even at the knees. When the loss is severe the unsteadiness that may have been present for years increases to render the patient incapable of walking in the dark and to need support even for walking in daylight. Motor weakness is slight or undetectable.

The degree of control of the diabetes seems to have little relevance to the onset of the neuropathy and there does not appear to be much evidence that maintaining ideal blood sugar levels improves the condition. Hypoglycaemic bouts should be avoided as far as possible since they may well hasten the onset or speed of progression of the neuropathy.

In a few cases, and especially in older men who have recently lost weight, a bilateral asymmetric weakness of the thigh muscles develops. There is pain in the front of the thighs, tenderness on compressing the quadriceps and obvious wasting. This condition is called diabetic amyotrophy and seems to be caused by involvement of multiple lumbar nerve roots.

A full and excellent review of the management of diabetes and its complications can be found in the British Medical Journal booklet *ABC of Diabetes.*

CHRONIC URAEMIA

Now that the patients with chronic uraemia are surviving for long periods with dialysis it has become obvious that one of the complications of the condition is a mixed peripheral neuropathy. It is said to affect about one-half of the patients and can be really quite severe. The combination of a sensory loss and weakness results in a severe unsteadiness that is not always restored by frequent and otherwise effective dialysis. Successful renal transplantation seems to result in a reversal of the neuropathy and a return to normal can be anticipated although it may be long delayed. The mechanism of the neuropathy is unclear although demyelination of the peripheral nerves is found on biopsy.

There may be other causes of unsteadiness in treated uraemics. Frequently they have been given courses of aminoglycoside antibiotics and these can insidiously or acutely damage the vestibular labyrinth of the inner ear. A slow loss often results in oscillopsia with the surroundings apparently moving about as the patient walks. This is described in more detail in Chapter 2. Asymmetric and rapid damage causes vertigo and this can be particularly distressing when it comes on in addition to the general malaise that attends the anaemia, the infections or treatment.

The handling of many drugs, a few of which cause a peripheral neuropathy, is impaired by poor renal function, and this must always be considered when prescribing, especially in the elderly.

DRUGS

Some of the drugs that cause a specific peripheral neuropathy as an unwanted side-effect are likely only to be used in specialised circumstances when the complication may be anticipated. Isoniazid used in the treatment of tuberculosis is the classic example as doses of more than 400 mg per day regularly cause paraesthesiae, burning feelings, and even mental changes in susceptible individuals. Alterations in pyridoxine metabolism are the cause and the neuropathy should be treated with 25 to 50 mg of pyridoxine per day.

Vincristine, used in the treatment of the acute leukaemias, lymphomas and some solid tumours of the breast and lung, rather commonly causes trouble with a peripheral and autonomic neuropathy. The peripheral effects are mainly sensory

195

and their onset should suggest reduction in the drug dose. If an obvious motor neuropathy develops it is probably wiser to withdraw the drug.

The use of gold injections in the treatment of rheumatoid arthritis can, amongst the many other problems occasionally cause a peripheral neuropathy.

The unsteadiness that results from these unwanted side-effects are usually recognised as such, since the drugs are often administered by specialist units. Nitrofurantoin however is commonly used in general practice for the treatment of uncomplicated urinary tract infections. If renal function is impaired with a glomerular filtration rate of less than 50 ml/min (equivalent to a serum creatinine of approximately 150 μmol/litre) then a peripheral neuropathy is commonly induced by this drug. Renal function declines with age and many elderly patients have a glomerular filtration rate of less than 50 ml/min which may not be reflected by raised serum creatinine levels. The prescription of nitrofurantoin should therefore be avoided in the elderly as its side-effects add to the slight unsteadiness caused by the general decline in the efficiency of the vestibular system and of visual acuity.

Conversely elderly patients with unsteadiness must be asked closely what medicines they take, and answers such as 'water tablets' not be accepted as meaning diuretics. If the tablets cannot be named perhaps they can be produced even if it means another visit. Stopping the nitrofurantoin is often just enough to reverse the unsteadiness and restore reasonable balance.

Recently allopurinol, used as mainstay treatment for gout, has been noted to cause a peripheral sensory neuropathy in patients with poor renal function and although not apparently a common complication it is reversible (Worth and Hussein 1985).

VITAMIN DEFICIENCIES

In the western world pure dietary deficiency of the B vitamins is rare, and those causes that do occur are nearly always in association with alcoholism. However failure of absorption of vitamin B_{12} can occur and present not as anaemia but as a progressive peripheral neuropathy. Tinglings in the feet and calves come first and progress to unpleasant burning sensations that extend further up the legs. The earliest detectable sign is loss of vibration sense in the feet and calves, and as time goes by, of joint position sense. Difficulty in walking with unsteadiness comes next, and Romberg's test becomes positive with obvious ataxia of the legs shown by the heel–shin test. Motor symptoms tend to arrive later but without treatment the weakness progresses to render the patient helpless. The condition rejoices under the name 'subacute combined degeneration of the cord', and is a diagnosis not to be missed. At the same time there are often mild central neurological effects with perhaps a loss of memory and poor concentration being ascribed to age or slight dementia.

The commonest cause of failure to absorb vitamin B_{12} is pernicious anaemia. This is rare in the young but the incidence rises progressively after the age of 35. Although ubiquitous, pernicious anaemia appears to be especially prevalent in people of northern European descent, and is typically found in those who are blue-eyed, well-built and given to premature greying of the hair. Many will be of blood group A, but there is no clear pattern of inheritance of the condition.

Normal absorption of vitamin B_{12} depends on the secretion of intrinsic factor by the parietal cells in the fundus of the stomach. In pernicious anaemia this secretion stops and the symptoms eventually develop as tissue levels of B_{12} fall. After total gastrectomy the same condition will of course arise and since the vitamin B_{12}/intrinsic factor complex is absorbed in the ileum, conditions that involve this region may also lead to an eventual deficiency. Coeliac disease, Crohn's disease or ileal bypass surgery are all examples. Some uptake of B_{12} by the intrinsic gut flora is usual but if there is an overgrowth as can occur in small bowel diverticula, or when ileal loops have been created by disease or at surgery, not enough B_{12} is available and the deficiency symptoms gradually occur.

The way to diagnose B_{12} deficiency is not to give an injection of B_{12} to see if the symptoms get better for this will completely destroy the value of any subsequent blood investigations. The formula of history, examination and investigations should be followed as ever. Symptoms of anaemia, which include lightheadedness, sometimes to be confused with unsteadiness, and a history of previous abdominal surgery may be helpful. The patient may have been treated in the past for Crohn's disease, or ulcerative colitis.

The examination reveals the signs of the peripheral neuropathy described above, but there may also be features of anaemia with, especially in those with pernicious anaemia, a lemonish tinge in a waxy, pale skin.

A full blood count usually shows anaemia, but in those with only the peripheral neuropathy, the haemoglobin is normal although a macrocytosis with abnormal red cell forms, and a reduction in the white cell count is found. Blood should be taken for assay of B_{12} and folate levels. Further specialised investigations will be needed to establish the definitive cause of the deficiency, and the extent of investigation varies from centre to centre. However once the deficiency has been confirmed it is reasonable to start replacement therapy, which, in those with pernicious anaemia or the post-gastrectomy cases, will need to be life-long.

Sometimes folic acid, alone or in combination with iron, is given to patients who have vague symptoms of anaemia, and perhaps a little unsteadiness in the hope that 'a vitamin tonic' will make them better. This is unwise because folic acid does not stop the progress of the neuropathy caused by B_{12} deficiency and may even make it worse. In addition, the anaemia may be masked, thereby confusing the correct diagnosis. With correct treatment the early neuropathies improve significantly but established motor loss rarely gets better. The mental changes recover only slowly.

NON-METASTATIC EFFECTS OF CANCER

Cancer can involve the nervous system directly, by way of metastatic deposits, or as has been recognised more recently by a process in which there is no direct involvement by the growth. These non-metastatic effects can produce a remarkable variety of neurological lesions (Brain and Norris 1965) which often precede the symptoms of the underlying cancer. Only a few per cent of cancer patients have any non-metastatic involvement of the nervous system and those with malignancies in the ovary and lung are most frequently troubled, whilst rectal and uterine cancers rarely cause problems.

The peripheral nerves can be involved by a pure sensory neuropathy with a rapidly progressive loss of vibration and joint position sense in the feet and legs. Skin sensation diminishes but power remains normal. There is initial pain then clumsiness and unsteadiness, and these symptoms usually precede the appearance of the cancer responsible for them. More commonly a mixed sensory and motor loss occurs. This begins again with aches and pains in the legs and then sensory loss and weakness develop. Cerebellar degeneration can also occur adding central ataxia to the sensorimotor ataxia in the legs. Surprisingly the condition often undergoes spontaneous remission even though the cancer is untreated.

Thus, when any unusual peripheral neuropathy makes its appearance and cannot be explained after the more common causes have been excluded, the presence of carcinoma should be suspected. Often however even an extensive search may fail to reveal the underlying growth and only time brings the correct diagnosis. No useful treatment has yet been found in these non-metastatic peripheral neuropathies.

HYPOTHYROIDISM

Just occasionally a peripheral neuropathy can arise before the more florid signs of hypothyroidism develop. It is a mainly sensory neuropathy that resembles that caused by any of the other conditions. The tendon reflexes however are often abnormal with the slow relaxation phase typical of the more advanced disease. Other symptoms can also present before the typical sluggishness, weight gain and sleepiness appear. Carpal tunnel syndrome, hoarseness, irregular or very heavy periods are additional features that may suggest the cause. About ten per cent of patients with idiopathic hypothyroidism will also have pernicious anaemia and, as well as performing thyroid function tests to establish the diagnosis, the serum B_{12} should be assayed if there is a peripheral neuropathy.

DAMAGE AND DISEASE IN THE SPINAL CORD

Compression of the spinal cord

Damage to the spinal cord can cause unsteadiness and difficulty in walking as power and sensation are lost from the legs. Frequently there is pain, and sometimes an additional disturbance of bladder and bowel function. Some patients will present as an emergency with a serious problem such as paralysis, pain or retention of urine. A catastrophe like this can be caused by direct trauma to the cord, a bleed into the cord, or sudden compression from collapse of a vertebra or protrusion of an intervertebral disc. These conditions do not concern us in a discussion of unsteadiness as it is the slowly progressive disorders that are likely to cause a disturbance of balance. A list of the commonest causes is given in Table 16.2.

The speed of onset of symptoms naturally varies with the specific cause, being slow with spinal tumours but more rapid with secondary carcinoma. In general the first symptoms are sensory, the commonest being pain radiating out in the distribution of one or more of the spinal nerves. These pains are usually most severe when caused by collapse of a vertebra, are frequently bad when a neurofibroma is present but are not so marked with a tumour growing within the cord.

The pains are often burning in quality and maybe made worse by bending or sudden movement. Compression of different sensory tracts within the cord gives rise to a range of other sensations. Numbness, coldness, heat, heaviness, a feeling that the leg is swollen or enclosed in a tight bandage can all be present. There can of course be localised pain and tenderness in the back at the site of the problem especially when there is malignant disease of the vertebral bodies.

Motor symptoms develop later and there is usually weakness,

Table 16.2: Conditions causing problems with the spinal cord

Disease of vertebral column

    2° carcinoma, esp. breast, thyroid, prostate, lung
    Cervical spondylosis
    Protrusion of intervertebral disc
    Tuberculous and other forms of oseitis
    1° tumours

Intravertebral causes of compression

    Outside the spinal cord
        Meningiomas
        Neurofibromas
    Within the spinal cord
        1° gliomas — mainly ependymomas
        Rarely 2° deposits

stiffness and unsteadiness. When the compression occurs below the cervical region of the cord, the motor symptoms are restricted to the legs. If the motor roots themselves or their cell bodies in the anterior horns of grey matter in the cord are compressed, a lower motor neurone type of lesion results with weakness, wasting, absent or diminished reflexes and fasciculation. Compression of the nerve fibres descending from the cerebral cortex via the corticospinal tracts to supply these anterior horn cells, results in an upper motor neurone type of lesion lower down. There is weakness, rigidity, increased reflexes and upgoing plantar responses (a positive Babinski sign) (Figure 16.1).

Thus, compression at one level can result in a lower motor neurone type of weakness to the muscles supplied by that

Figure 16.1: Highly schematic and simplified diagram of some of the effects of damage to the spinal cord. On the left hand side external pressure is causing motor symptoms and producing a lower motor neurone lesion at the site of the lesion with upper motor neurone signs further down. On the right hand side a further lesion within the cord is predominantly affecting sensory pathways. When the ascending dorsal columns are involved proprioception, vibration, light pressure and touch are involved and this would be typical of external compression from a neuroma of the dorsal sensory root. With the lesion shown the cross spinothalamic pathways are involved and pain and temperature sensation are involved. Various combinations are usually found in practice.

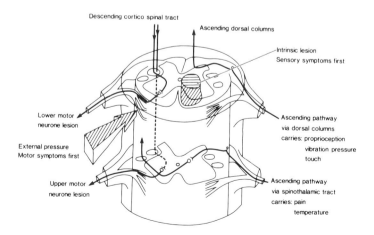

segment and an upper motor neurone weakness to muscles supplied by nerves arising lower down the cord.

Later on the bladder and bowel can be affected with difficulty in passing urine, urinary retention and constipation.

If the patient is carefully examined some sensory loss can usually be found, although the extent may not bear much relationship to the level at which cord damage has occurred. The tendon reflexes should also be tested and can be useful although interpretation may be difficult. A symmetrical absence of reflexes can be found in normal people, but asymmetric loss is abnormal. If the missing reflex can be elicited with reinforcement during the test then it is less likely to be abnormal. Symmetrically very brisk reflexes are also remarkably common in health as are a few beats of clonus and an obviously exaggerated unilateral reflex is needed to be of any help in diagnosis. The levels of the various reflexes are given in Table 16.3. Small differences in tone are almost impossible to assess, and by the time the limbs are flaccid or rigid the diagnosis is usually not in doubt. The same can be said for the plantar reflex which is usually equivocal when you would most like it to be definitely positive or negative to help with the diagnosis. Autonomic changes with excessive sweating below the level of the lesion can sometimes be detected and when found are helpful in adding to the weight of the clinical evidence.

Plain radiographs of the spine can help when collapse or erosion of the vertebral bodies is found but even severe degenerative changes with loss of disc space and association osteophyte formation is not helpful as this is such a common finding in the population without symptoms of cord compression. Further specialised examination of symptomatic patients is necessary because although many of the conditions are untreat-

Table 16.3: Localisation of tendon reflexes

Reflex	Spinal segment	Peripheral nerve
Biceps	Cervical 5, 6	Musculo-cutaneous
Triceps	Cervical 6, 7	Radial
Supinator	Cervical 5, 6	Radial
Finger flexors	Cervical 7, 8	Median and ulnar
Knee	Lumbar 2–4	Femoral
Ankle	Sacral 1, 2	Sciatic

able a few can be cured and timely surgical intervention may prevent the disaster of a profound paraplegia.

Compression of the spinal cord needs to be distinguished from disseminated sclerosis and less commonly from motor neurone disease and spinal syphilis.

Disseminated sclerosis

This condition has been described in Chapter 14 as a cause of vertigo following brainstem involvement. The spinal cord may also become involved and several clinical pictures have been described. A gradual onset of weakness in one or both legs is common, a sudden weakness less so. Together these two presentations form one of the major causes of weakness of the legs in young adults. Sometimes sensory symptoms are the presenting feature with 'numbness' spreading from feet to waist developing over a few days and associated with difficulty in walking. These symptoms persist for a few days or weeks before remission occurs. The examination in all these forms of presentation will usually reveal rigidity, exaggerated reflexes and sometimes upgoing plantars, whilst characteristically vibration sense is absent.

If any of these complaints are the first presenting features of disseminated sclerosis then differentiation from cord compression may not be possible without a myelogram or computerised tomography. Resolution of the weakness, numbness or unsteadiness suggests that DS is the cause of the problem as cord compression tends to progress relentlessly. A good history of any of the other features of DS helps in confirming the diagnosis, but should the symptoms persist then a referral for investigation should be made because some other treatable pathology involving the spinal cord might just co-exist.

Motor neurone disease

Motor neurone disease results from degenerative changes most marked in the anterior horn cells of the spinal cord, in the motor nuclei of the lower brainstem and in the corticospinal tracts. The result is a progressive mixture of upper and lower motor neurone symptoms and signs. The exact clinical pattern depends on the extent and the site of involvement and so a number of classifications have developed but are not important here. The cause is unknown but the disease is one of late and middle life, frequently starting between the ages of 50 and 70, although onset in the 30s and 40s can occur. The condition usually involves the hands and arms first with cramp-like pains, weakness, stiffness, clumsiness, wasting and fasciculation, although the same pattern can occur first in the legs and present as unsteadiness. Although there is weakness there is no sensory loss and this finding helps during the early stages to distinguish motor neurone disease from cord compression.

As the motor nuclei of the lower brainstem become involved a progressive bulbar palsy develops. The tongue becomes shrunken and wrinkled and shows fasciculation (XII nerve). The muscles of the lips (VII) the extrinsic muscles of the palate then pharynx and larynx (IX and X) become involved so that swallowing becomes difficult, the speech slurred and regurgitation and finally aspiration occur. Although there is no effective treatment, continuing care and support is important especially when the symptoms of bulbar palsy develop as surgery may be necessary to help with the problems of swallowing and aspiration.

Spinal syphilis — tabes dorsalis

Syphilis affecting the spinal cord comes in two distinct categories: that involving the meninges and blood vessels and that involving the spinal cord itself. Meningo-vascular syphilis is particularly rare, but patients with the second form of involvement have tabes dorsalis and may present with unsteadiness, although this condition is also uncommon. Patients with tabes tend to deny having had a primary chancre or any of the secondary manifestations and this is not just shame or embarrassment but probably a different reaction to the spirochaete. The sensory spinal nerves (the dorsal roots) atrophy, as do their continuations, the ascending afferent tracts (the posterior columns) of the spinal cord. The lower portions of the cord tend to be involved first, and the onset of symptoms is usually gradual and insidious.

When the lumbar regions of the cord are involved, pain is the most characteristic early symptom, usually in the form of stabbing 'lightning' shocks in the legs. These tend to be localised to one spot and each attack lasts but a few seconds. The pains can be restricted to one site or shift from place to place. They can of course be found in other parts of the body when other sections of the cord are involved. Paraesthesiae may occur with the feet feeling numb or cold, or the patient feeling as if he is walking on cotton wool.

On sensory testing, vibration sense is usually the first to go. Pain cannot be elicited from the muscles and tendons in response to forceful squeezing, whilst, surprisingly, skin sensation stays intact. With this combination of sensory loss, unsteadiness develops and is of course worse in the dark, or on turning rapidly. As a more florid ataxia develops, the patient walks with a wide base, his feet are lifted high up and stamped down. Finally a walking stick is not enough to enhance the somatosensory input and the patient needs support. Romberg's test becomes positive early on and the performance of the heel-shin test impossible.

When the sacral roots are involved, which can be before or after the lumbar roots, bladder and bowel symptoms and impotence occur.

The pupils are usually abnormal at sometime during the course of protracted tabes, although the full-blown Argyll-Robertson pupil — where the reaction to light is impaired then lost whilst that to accommodation is retained — is a late sign.

Occasionally the onset of tabes is rapid and Oliver Sacks is his excellent monograph 'The man who mistook his wife for a hat' eloquently describes such a presentation:

A patient, Charles D., was referred to us for stumbling, falls and vertigo — there had been unfounded suspicions of labyrinthine disorder. It was evident on closer questioning that what he experienced was not vertigo at all, but a flutter of ever-changing positional illusions — suddenly the floor seemed further, then suddenly nearer, it pitched, it jerked, it tilted — in his own words 'like a ship in heavy seas'. In consequence he found himself lurching and pitching, unless he looked down at his feet. Vision was necessary to show him the true position of his feet and the floor — feel had become grossly unstable and misleading — but sometimes even vision was overwhelmed by feel, so that the floor and his feet looked frightening and shifting.

205

We soon ascertained that he was suffering from the acute onset of tabes — and (in consequence of dorsal root involvement) from a sort of sensory delirium of rapidly fluctuating 'proprioceptive illusions'. Everyone is familiar with the classical end-stage of tabes, in which there may be virtual proprioceptive 'blindness' for the legs. Have readers encountered this intermediate stage — of positional phantoms or illusions — due to an acute (and reversible) tabetic delirium? (Oliver Sacks 1985, courtesy Gerald Duckworth and Co.).

The specific diagnosis of syphilis is made by serological testing — the FTA (Abs.) being the most specific. Treatment is with penicillin and steroids and is best undertaken by a specialist unit.

17

The Cerebral Cortex and Psyche

The final chapter on the conditions that can cause dizziness describes some specific problems where drugs or disease directly affects function, but also contains some ill-defined entities that have ended up here since the pathology is unknown and they are therefore difficult to place in any other category; drop attacks are probably the best example of this problem.

DRUGS AFFECTING THE CENTRAL VESTIBULAR PATHWAYS

Any drug affecting the central processing of incoming vestibular information or the resulting output to the skeletal and ocular muscles is likely to affect balance, with a variety of forms of dizziness being possible. This is usually not a problem in the young, but with increasing age and an inability to 'handle' the drug optimally, compensation for the side-effects of the drug is inadequate and the patients feel dizzy, especially if they are anaemic, drink too much alcohol or take other drugs which can interact. The effect is usually unsteadiness, but momentary bouts of vertigo can result from rapid head movement or positional change. Under the influence of drugs a sudden change in the visual field or something like a stream of cars passing rapidly by, can trigger one or two seconds worth of vertigo, unsteadiness or the non-specific symptoms of giddiness. The drugs most likely to be associated with these complaints are set out in Table 17.1, and withdrawal of the offending drug, or reduction in its dose may just be enough to convert an unsteady individual into one who is mobile and feels safe.

Table 17.1: Drugs affecting central pathways and causing dizziness

Analgesics:	Narcotic analgesics:
	Morphine
	Dextropropoxyphenone
	Codeine
	Dihydrocodeine
	Paracetamol
	Pentazocine
Psychotropics:	Tricyclic antidepressants
	Phenothiazines, e.g. chlorpromazine
	Benzodiazepines, e.g. diazepam
Anticonvulsants:	Carbamazepine
	Clonazepam
	Primidone
	Phenytoin
Anti-Parkinsonians:	Benzhexol
	L-Dopa
Hypnotics:	Barbiturates

ALTERATIONS IN THE BLOOD SUPPLY TO THE BRAIN

Syncope is a transient reduction of consciousness. The conditions that cause the faint can also give rise to feelings of light-headedness without progressing to the completed attack when the symptom, if not the diagnosis, is clear. The light-headedness may be accompanied by other features such as difficulty in thinking, blurred vision and weakness which are general symptoms, related to any such attack, and by slightly more specific symptoms such as pallor, a clammy skin, sweating and nausea which give a clue to the cause. Syncope is really very common and results either from a transitory impairment in cerebral blood flow, or a reduction of oxygen, glucose or carbon dioxide below that level needed to maintain function. In this section the more common conditions and their diagnosis are described.

The common faint

The common faint, or vasovagal attack, is by far the most frequent cause of fainting and those that do not quite lose consciousness often complain of the light-headedness that accompanies the other symptoms. The attack is brought on by sudden emotional stress associated with fear, anxiety or pain. It is common in fit young people and even a smell or a sight can induce the chain of reactions that lead to a fall in cerebral perfusion. There is initial pallor, nausea and sweating, followed by dilation of the pupils, yawning, deep breathing and a marked slowing of the pulse. During this phase light-headedness is nearly universal, and will be the complaint if the attack fails to progress.

Fortunately most young people appear to lose the fainting tendency as years go by, probably because 'vagal tone' declines. Usually the picture is clear when the history is taken and simple reassurance may be all that is needed to quell anxiety. However spontaneous attacks without any obvious initiating factor — the sight of blood, the smell of hospitals — for example require a thorough examination and the distinction from the aura of epilepsy or Stokes-Adams attacks may be difficult.

Chronic orthostatic hypotension

A failing autonomic nervous system has, as one of its manifestations an inability of the peripheral blood vessels to compensate for postural changes. Pooling of blood occurs in the legs and guts when any individual is lying down, but when a patient with an autonomic insufficiency stands there is an immediate and sharp fall in blood pressure with light-headedness but no pallor, sweating or nausea. Associated features in the history are impotence, difficulty with passing urine because of bladder dysfunction, and loss of sweating in the feet and calves.

During an attack the pulse stays the same and the condition is easily diagnosed by having the patient lie flat on the couch or bed for five to ten minutes, at the end of which time his blood pressure and pulse are taken. He is then stood up quickly and the blood pressure and pulse retaken after ten or twenty seconds.

Diabetes and syphilis can cause the autonomic neuropathy and should be excluded. The drug history must be carefully taken since alpha-adrenergic sympathetic blocking agents (tolazoline, phenoxybenzamine and even chlorpromazine to some extent), adrenergic neurone blockers (guanethidine, bethanidine, methyldopa) and vasodilators in all shape and size can have postural hypotension and dizziness as a side-effect. However having excluded these, and the rare form of Parkinsonism that is associated with postural hypotension (Shy-Drager syndrome) the way is open to call the condition idiopathic orthostatic hypotension. Since there is no known cause there is no cure but effective treatment can be provided by the provision of 'antigravity stockings' which prevent or restrict the venous pooling in the legs.

Stokes-Adams attacks

Giovanni Battista Morgagni's (1682–1771) major work *The seats and causes of disease* which was published when he was 80, gives the first clear account of heart block and its association with convulsive attacks (Morgagni 1769). A paper published by Thomas Spens in 1793 contains the first account of heart block written by a British physician and precedes that of William Stokes by 53 years and that of Robert Adams by 48 years. Such are the fortunes of life however that Stokes and Adams now have their names attached to the condition.

The patient has a persistently slow pulse in the region of 40 or less, which is secondary to disordered atrio-ventricular conduction. Spontaneous episodes of asystole, ventricular fibrillation or tachycardia occur when consciousness can be impaired. If the disordered rhythm persists long enough consciousness is lost and convulsions can occur. William Stokes, who was a prolific writer, in his paper 'Observations on Some Cases of a Permanently Low Pulse' (Stokes 1846) noted that one of his patients was able to ward off the attacks 'by a peculiar manoeuvre; as soon as he perceives symptoms of the approaching attack he directly turns on his hands and knees keeping his head low and by this means, he says, he often averts what otherwise would end in an attack'.

The slow pulse, an abnormal electrocardiogram and 24-hour cardiac monitoring now allows definitive diagnosis and provides a firm basis for treatment with some form of pacemaker.

Other cardiac problems can also cause bouts of altered cerebral perfusion with light-headedness. Many are secondary to previous infarction and presumably result from alterations in cardiac rhythm, but one not to miss in aortic stenosis, since light-headedness or fainting on exertion is a bad prognostic symptom, and may be a forerunner to sudden death. The blood pressure in these patients is usually normal and hypertension with a systolic pressure over 200 mm Hg virtually excludes the condition. The peripheral arterial pulses characteristically rise slowly and on listening to the heart a pan-systolic 'diamond shaped' murmur is heard best down the right costal margin with extension up into the neck. The decision to be made with these patients is to their suitability for aortic valve replacement and they should be referred to the appropriate cardiothoracic centre.

In a few older patients, and especially in those with cardio-vascular disease, the carotid sinus response is particularly effective in slowing the pulse and dropping the blood pressure, with resulting light-headedness. The carotid sinus lies at the bifurcation of the common carotid which is at the level of the upper border of the thyroid cartilage and occasionally light-headedness can be brought on by turning the head, especially when a tight collar is being worn. The effects are not accompanied by pallor, nausea or sweating and can sometimes be elicited by very gently massaging the relevant area of the neck on one side only. Great care should be taken to avoid occluding the carotid as strokes have sometimes resulted from this manoeuvre. Carotid sinus massage can be useful however in a patient who suddenly develops rapid atrial fibrillation and the procedure with electro-cardiographic control can bring about return to sinus rhythm.

Cough and micturition effects

Following a bout of vigorous coughing or even side-splitting laughter transient light-headedness can occur and may in some instances progress to a faint. The light-headedness following coughing is usually found in men with chronic bronchitis, but as with that which follows laughing, the exact mechanism is unclear. It has been suggested that the presence of an intra-cranial tumour or stenosis of one of the major cerebral blood vessels enhances the effect when the light-headedness is accompanied by other symptoms such as twitching, tingling or numbness in an arm or leg. Such cases should be referred for neurological assessment but in the vast majority without these additional symptoms little can be done to overcome the light-headedness other than rigorously treating the chest condition

211

after excluding bronchogenic carcinoma.

Light-headedness during or just after passing urine is usually reported by men who, having drunk too much beer during the evening get up at night to empty their bladder. The combination of the peripheral vasodilation caused by alcohol, standing and rapidly emptying a distended bladder brings on a faintness through a variety of mechanisms, but the same effect can be seen in an innocent patient with acute retention of urine who has just been catheterised and all the urine let out at once, by mistake.

Hyperventilation syndrome

Overbreathing nearly always results from acute anxiety when the effects of hyperventilation might be mingled with sensations arising from an associated panic attack. The whole collection of symptoms usually starts with the patient feeling closed in and surrounded, with a tightness in the chest and throat. She feels as if she is about to suffocate and may remember sighing deeply although the overbreathing is rarely recalled or admitted. As the overbreathing continues, the patient feels dissociated or out of contact with reality, and may have a sense of impending doom. Light-headedness, giddiness, unsteadiness and shakes develop and are often the major complaint. Tinglings around the lips, numbness and coldness of the hands and feet are typical accompanying complaints, as are palpitations.

The light-headedness and unsteadiness settle along with most of the other complaints as the attack settles, but the sense of unreality can, and often does, persist for many hours, and the bouts of hyperventilation can recur many times during the day.

Why hyperventilation can cause all these effects is not clear but the symptoms can usually be reproduced exactly by getting the patient to overbreathe when she can be shown that it is this and not any serious underlying disease that is causing the problem. She should also be shown that rebreathing into a paper or polythene bag will rapidly abolish the symptoms as will breath-holding. Very occasionally this reassurance is enough to break the cycle of panic attack causing hyperventilation resulting in fear of the symptoms produced by the hyperventilation causing further panic. More often the underlying anxiety needs evaluation and treatment.

Hypoglycaemic attacks

Failure to supply the brain with enough glucose causes weakness, faintness and confusion — all of which are often lumped together and called dizzy, giddy, light-headed and so on. The patient may have noticed the rapid improvement that occurs by eating something sweet when the symptoms start to develop. If the patient is a diabetic then the diagnosis is often simple and his medication or insulin dosages should be carefully checked, and either these or his eating habits readjusted. Several drugs interact with the hypoglycaemic agents potentiating or antagonising their effects and so the patient should be asked closely if they are taking, or have just stopped taking, any other medicines (see Table 17.2).

The contraceptive pill is often forgotten by the patient to be a medicine and so the patient should be asked specifically whether she has stopped taking 'the pill'.

In those patients who are not diabetic the light-headedness may come on after a heavy meal. In those patients who have had extensive gastric resection, or a procedure such as vagotomy and pyloroplasty which hastens gastric emptying this is called the 'dumping syndrome'. Within half an hour of a large

Table 17.2: Interactions with antidiabetic drugs

General interaction with oral agents and insulin

Potentiate the hypoglycaemic effects
  Alcohol
  Beta-adrenergic blockers
  Mono-amine oxidase inhibitors

Antagonise the hypoglycaemic effects
  Corticosteroids
  Diazoxide
  Diuretics: bumetanide, frusemide, thiazides
  Oral contraceptives

Specific interactions with the sulphonylureas (chlorpropamide, tolbutamide)
  Chloramphenicol
  Clofibrate
  Co-trimoxazole
  Miconazole
  Phenylbutazone
  Sulphinpyrazone

meal there is a feeling of fullness, intense drowsiness and fatigue. In addition, there may be some vascular symptom with palpitations, pallor or sweating. The individual may even have to lie down whilst the early symptoms, which are probably secondary to hyperglycaemia, pass. The late symptoms that arise an hour or more after the meal has finished, are a result of a reactive hypoglycaemia that has occurred because of an over-production of insulin. The typical hypoglycaemic symptoms are accentuated or brought on by exercise and can be reproduced by an injection of short-acting soluble insulin.

The dumping syndrome following surgery frequently settles with time but can be helped by advising the patient to replace a carbohydrate-rich diet with one containing more fats and meats, which appear to delay gastric emptying. Taking glucose when 'late' symptoms are present will abolish them but is probably not a method to be recommended, unless all else fails.

Hypoglycaemic attacks can also occur without previous gastric surgery in tense individuals who eat high carbohydrate diets. The effects resemble the late symptoms described for the dumping syndrome and can usually be managed by altering the diet.

Hypoglycaemic attacks following exercise and unrelated to meal-times can of course be caused by pure or simple starvation and may occur in boxers, jockeys, or even dedicated dieters who are trying to lose weight. More rarely insulin-producing islet cell tumours of the pancreas do the same but in these the early morning, fasting blood sugar level is often low.

DROP ATTACKS

A drop attack is an unexpected fall that usually occurs when walking, or standing, but never when sitting. The patient is nearly always female and often in middle age. The fall is surprisingly nearly always forwards and the patients therefore frequently sustain grazed knees, Colle's or scaphoid fractures, or injuries to the face. Consciousness, if lost at all, is only for a split second during the fall itself, and the sufferers quickly scramble to their feet again, often feeling stupid or highly embarrassed. The lack of warning, the injuries caused and the feeling of being silly often makes the patient fearful of going out alone, and may severely restrict normal living, or induce an anxiety state. Drop attacks appear to occur more commonly around the menopause or in premenopausal women during the premenstrual week although the association is difficult to establish firmly. Otherwise the attacks are irregular and cannot be predicted.

In a very few of those who suffer from drop attacks there is some underlying or additional neurological disorder. Epilepsy is at the top of the list, along with cerebrovascular disease, but occasionally the condition is found when myopathies or neuropathies cause weakness in the legs and rarely with tumours in the third ventricle. These conditions may either cause the drop attacks or by chance occur concurrently. However in the great majority of women with drop attacks there is no detectable pathology and the decision that needs to be made is how far to investigate them to exclude the other uncommon conditions. An otherwise blameless history and a normal neurological examination will be enough for many physicians, but others would like to see a normal electroencephalogram and perhaps a normal CT or magnetic resonance scan of the head before labelling the condition as idiopathic. The decision depends on many factors, one of which is easy access to the newer imaging facilities.

Treatment of drop attacks, whether idiopathic or associated with other conditions, is unsatisfactory, although once the associated conditions have been excluded, the positive confirmation that there is no sinister disease at work is often reassuring and may help to restore confidence. Fortunately many women stop having drop attacks after a few years, although this is of little comfort to them if they have just sustained a serious facial injury.

EPILEPSY

'Epilepsy' is a blanket word that encompasses all the features that result from transient misbehaviour of the brain caused by excessive neuronal discharge. The condition is common with a prevalence of about 0.5 per cent in the general population and the effects can be focal when it seems that one portion of the brain is affected, or generalised when most of the brain becomes involved. Frequently an initial focal discharge spreads so rapidly to become generalised that the distinction is unclear. It is customary to divide the epilepsies into idiopathic or acquired.

215

The idiopathic group, which form about three-quarters of the total have a strong genetic association with the relatives of a sufferer having six to ten times greater risk of epilepsy than the rest of the population. Acquired epilepsy results from a structural disorder in the brain. The list of causes is almost endless but congenital conditions such as haemangiomas, maternal rubella and birth asphyxia are common. Later on in life infections, especially those from the ear and the sinuses, head injury, primary and secondary brain tumours and, in the older age groups, cerebrovascular disease, all make a contribution.

Epilepsy can, of course, present in many forms and those with an aura, unconsciousness and a fit do not concern us here. However, the epilepsy may consist of the aura alone as the focal discharge fails to spread from its site or origin. Depending on the location of the focal discharge the symptoms can include dizziness. Lesions in the temporal lobe occasionally cause vertigo, but more often the sensation perceived from lesions here and elsewhere are less specific and without the illusion of movement. Giddiness serves to cover the peculiar sensations or disordered balance, of fear of falling, or disorientation and so on, and as such is frequently used by patients. Of course there may be other components in the aura with anxiety and a peculiar epigastric sensation welling up into the throat being common. Unpleasant smells or tastes can develop and the patient often feels dreamy and confused. Although the temporal lobe is often the site or origin of such a collection of symptoms, focal lesions in the frontal and occipital lobes can also produce giddiness as part of the aura although it seems likely that this is caused by secondary effects on the temporal lobe and limbic system.

The aura may progress to unconsciousness and collapse. If giddiness or vertigo has been part of the aura then it, rather than the unconsciousness, may be blamed for the fall. It is therefore important to determine from a friend or observer, the sequence of events and the occurrence of any loss of consciousness, since this feature indicates that the brain rather than the labyrinth is at fault.

When epilepsy is the cause of dizziness the diagnosis is often difficult. In females the attacks may occur in a fixed relationship to their menstrual cycle although not every month. They may only occur during the menopause and stop after ovulation has finally ceased. They may be made worse, or improve during pregnancy. A careful personal and family history may help separate the idiopathic from the acquired variety, but the onset of attacks in later life suggests that there might be disease elsewhere so that the symptoms relating to the common sites of origin of primary disease should be carefully pursued. The ears, nose and sinuses must not be forgotten in the hunt for the source of infection or embolus.

Between attacks the neurological examination usually fails to disclose significant abnormalities, especially in the idiopathic group. Temporal lobe lesions may however have an associated visual field defect as the lower fibres of the optic radiation sweep through this region. The result is an upper quadrant visual loss on the same side as the lesion (an upper homonymous quadrantic anopsia): with a tumour or an abscess arising from the disease in the mastoid, this defect is progressive, but if caused by a vascular episode the visual loss tends to improve as time passes.

Another early effect of a lesion in the upper part of the temporal lobe (the superior temporal gyrus) is a nominal dysphasia. This is a difficulty in specifically naming familiar objects although an appreciation of what the object does and a command of speech is retained. Thus, when one so affected is shown a watch and asked to say what it is, he will say that it is something used to tell the time and is held on the wrist by a strap. At a later examination when asked to name the strap of the watch, he may say that it is a band used to hold a watch to the wrist. The words 'watch' and 'strap' have not been lost from the vocabulary, nor is speech or thinking altered; the loss is in applying specific names, and when found is a valuable clue to disease in this region.

The general examination may reveal disease in the ears, nose, lungs or circulation and each should be pursued. At this stage referral to a neurologist for more specialised investigations is probably wise. A sleeping electroencephalogram is useful to detect temporal lobe abnormalities in the idiopathic group as the discharge pattern seems to be enhanced in the majority of adult sufferers when asleep. A CT or magnetic resonance scan may help to pick out a focal lesion.

The management of epilepsy is beyond the scope of this book but adequate control should eliminate the aura and its associated dizziness.

RELATIONSHIP OF DIZZINESS TO THE MENSTRUAL CYCLE

Anyone dealing with dizzy female patients will soon come to recognise that the symptoms are frequently made worse at certain specific times in the menstrual cycle, or develop or are exacerbated by the menopause. Pregnancy can also have an effect in either worsening or improving vestibular symptoms. This feature has already been noted in earlier sections on drop attacks and epilepsy but is also true for the vertigo that arises from ear disease and for the unsteadiness that may occur whilst compensation is taking place after labyrinthine or central vestibular damage. The severe attacks of vertigo that accompany Ménière's disease may have settled as the disease burns itself out, only to be reawakened during the menopause as bouts of vertigo or episodes of unsteadiness. By the same mechanism, the symptoms of an earlier, perhaps long-forgotten bout of vestibular neuronitis which left deranged, but compensated labyrinthine function, can recur during the menopause as unsteadiness or momentary flashes of vertigo.

The clinical evidence is difficult to deny but the mechanism is unknown, and, in general, attempts at hormonal replacement therapy during the menopause or the normal menstrual cycle have been unsuccessful in ridding the patient of symptoms. Many women however do feel generally better with specific hormonal therapy during the menopause and may be able to tolerate the unpleasant symptoms of dizziness, or dispense with the vestibular sedatives that are often prescribed.

Attacks of migraine are frequently related to the menstrual cycle and are thought to result from the physiological withdrawal of circulating oestrogen (Somerville 1975). Oral oestrogen therapy in these cases has not been very helpful but recent trials with percutaneous oestradiol administration have yielded promising results (de Lignieres, Vincens, Mauvais-Jarvis, Mas, Touboul and Bousser 1986) in abolishing or reducing the headache. Perhaps this will be a useful advance that, if confirmed, might just be applicable to those with menstrual vertigo.

The menstrual cycle or menopause is not, however, an excuse for relegating symptoms of dizziness to the status of 'something caused by the hormones'. This is especially so if there is no previous history of vestibular disorder. Many women are particularly distressed, when in addition to the expected menopausal symptoms they develop problems with balance and will fear something serious. A very few will have an underlying cause that needs treatment, and for this reason alone, all should be managed by having a good history taken and a thorough examination performed.

THE PSYCHE

Any, but the most stoic of individuals, struck by bouts of vertigo, prolonged episodes or feelings of light-headedness or giddiness are likely to have their confidence undermined, become anxious or fearful that there is major disease inside their head, and if the condition persists, become depressed by the interference caused to their life-style. Such reactions are easily understood and can be managed by treating the condition that causes the dizziness, by giving psychological support whilst the condition improves, and perhaps sometimes even providing medication in the form of short courses of the minor tranquillisers or even antidepressants. The vestibular exercises described in the next chapter, not only enhance central compensation for damaged vestibular pathways, but also provide a form of psychotherapy by re-establishing confidence and allowing verbal expression of fears and anxieties, especially in group therapy.

Dizziness causing psychiatric upset is thus one side of the coin but the reverse with psychiatric disorder causing dizziness also holds, although it may be much more difficult to evaluate. Many studies have shown that anxiety, depression and some of the personality disorders commonly cause physical symptoms of which dizziness, in all its forms is a particularly, if not the most, common complaint.

Anxiety

Anxiety is a normal and universal emotion, essential for effective living. It is generally an unpleasant sensation and is usually a feeling of something awful about to happen. It is not usually related to an actual threat — for this sensation would be called fear — but if there is a threat of some sort then the anxiety

219

produced is out of proportion to the minor nature of the actual threat. Along with the sensation of anxiety there is usually some physical discomfort. Many people have anxious personality traits and tend to feel anxious about things all the time without any major disturbance of day to day living.

Normal anxiety may be experienced before exams, after bereavement or divorce, and is usually tolerated by individuals as they recognise this as a response to an acute stress, and many know that a certain level of anxiety helps them cope with the problem.

Pathological anxiety symptoms arise when a person complains of having the feelings of anxiety or its physical manifestations more frequently, more severely or more persistently than he or she can tolerate, and it is this that sends him to the doctor with either the psychological or physical symptoms.

The patient with an anxiety neurosis presents with a cluster of symptoms centred on anxiety, the source of which is obscure or not easily understood. Dizziness is a very common major complaint and the diagnosis of an anxiety state depends on the association of the other symptoms which together with the dizziness make up the psychological and physical manifestations of excessive anxiety. Common additional symptoms are apprehension, inattention, difficulty in concentrating, fears of losing control, of impending disaster and dissociation from the world about them. Physical symptoms include sweating, tremor, chest pains, palpitations, a lump in the throat, tinglings and a dry mouth.

The sensation of an imminent loss of control, which is perhaps the most threatening feeling, can result in a panic attack with subsequent hyperventilation and the additional symptoms, including loss of consciousness described earlier in the chapter.

The anxiety may present as 'high level' anxiety lasting for hours or days during which time dizziness can be a prominent physical feature and persist through the attack or develop or be made worse by intervening panic attacks. Occasionally the anxiety can become chronic with persisting disabling unsteadiness or giddiness.

In developed countries anxiety neuroses seem to be particularly common, and depending on how the condition is defined affects perhaps two to four per cent of the population. The figure increases dramatically when the population sampled is that attending a medical clinic. Anxiety states are found predominantly in younger adults and whilst there is an excess of female sufferers in general practice, the sex ratio appears to be about equal in patients hospitalised for the condition. Mild or moderate anxiety states probably remit within a few months in the majority of cases whilst some go on to become chronic sufferers.

In many of the patients with an acute anxiety state the condition has been triggered by some recent event. This happening may be major and obvious or be minor and the enormity of the reaction ill-understood by the doctor. Nevertheless in previously stable individuals struck by dizziness resulting from excessive anxiety the condition can often be helped by reassurance and explanation that nothing awful is going to happen. Frequently this may be enough, but sometimes there will be the need to prescribe small doses of minor tranquillisers or beta adrenergic blockers, whilst the patients recover spontaneously.

In chronic anxiety induced by the environment and 'stress', the problem is more difficult. Some things may be remediable: the drunken spouse, the wife beater, the wayward child, may just be factors that can be changed, but unemployment, debt, poor housing are all unfortunate facts of life that it is often impossible for the individual doctor to alter. Here, counselling and assistance by the social workers should be enlisted, after the patient has been examined and reassured that there is no physical disease at work. Treatment with small doses of minor tranquillisers or betablockers may help the patients through bad patches.

Long lasting, low grade anxiety with episodes of giddiness laid on top of a generalised feeling of dissociation is particularly difficult to manage, and the temptation to prescribe large amounts of tranquillisers or vestibular sedatives should be strongly resisted. Formal psychiatric help may need to be requested but long-term studies suggest that only about one-half of this group recover or improve substantially.

Depression

Depression forms part of the collection of conditions called the affective disorders, and although some cases result from stress the cause in the majority is ill-understood, and the classification therefore tenuous. Nevertheless, three major groups can be

221

loosely defined under the cover of the term affective disorder. These three are psychotic depression, neurotic depression and mania. At present there are major trans-Atlantic differences as to whether the terms neurosis and psychosis should be used, but for ease of description and for want of better names they will be retained here.

Psychotic depression is also called endogenous depression as there is no obvious precipitating cause, although some psychiatrists feel that some 'event' can always be found if looked for carefully enough. Psychotic depression tends to arise in middle and later life in individuals who were previously stable and normal, although there is frequently a strong family history of depression. A persistent, sad, despairing mood, quite different from normal unhappiness is the underlying feature. Mood swings, far greater than those found in normal individuals are common as are hallucinations, which are usually auditory or visual. Feelings of inadequacy, guilt and uselessness develop and both thinking and functioning may be impaired so that the patient appears demented. An associated physical upset is common with anorexia, weight loss, loss of libido and alterations in the menstrual cycle.

Sometimes physical symptoms are the major presenting feature with the feelings of depression being relegated to a minor or background role. This state of affairs is termed masked depression and patients often present with vertigo or giddiness. On proper questioning, however, the patient will often report an 'undefined malaise ... a fear of rupture of the state of equilibrium' (Lopez Ibor 1972) and feelings of inadequacy and worthlessness on delving deeper. Bouts of depression may figure in the past history. After a neurologic and otologic examination has failed to show any underlying disorder, and a firm diagnosis of a masked depression has been made, the decision has to be made as to whether the patient should be referred for formal psychiatric assessment or whether initial treatment by the general practitioner or physician, with one of the many antidepressants should be attempted.

Neurotic or reactive depression occurs most typically in young adults in response to stress. This 'stress' may be seemingly quite trivial and has led many observers to suggest that the sufferers have an inadequate personality. Nevertheless, the despair is of the same quality as in a psychotic depression and is often associated with anxiety. Thinking is not disordered nor are bodily functions, and hallucinations are rare. Feelings of guilt and unworthiness are uncommon and the patient tends to blame others for his or her predicament. Dizziness is also rare in this group, unless brought on by the accompanying anxiety. Often the condition is self-limiting but antidepressant drugs and formal psychiatric assistance may be needed especially if there are suicidal thoughts.

Agoraphobia

Fear is a universal part of our existence, rather like anxiety, and in the same way can become overwhelming and handicap the sufferer when the condition is called a phobia. This morbid fear is disproportionate to the stimulus, cannot be explained away and leads to avoidance of the feared object or situation (Marks 1969). Anxiety and panic attacks frequently coexist with the phobia and may make the clinical picture difficult to untangle. Agoraphobia is the commonest of the phobias and is found most frequently in women in early adult life. The problems often start after a major happening such as bereavement, marriage or miscarriage or following a serious illness. The over-whelming sentiment is a fear of leaving a safe place such as home, and this becomes a fear of the outside world, the things in it or the situations that can crop up. The phobia often manifests itself as giddiness, or a fear of falling and close questioning as to the circumstances surrounding the attack usually leads to the correct diagnosis.

Treatment is more difficult than diagnosis, but there are several self-help groups for agoraphobics who attempt to wean the sufferer back into the community one step at a time. Various other forms of behaviour therapy have been tried although the generalised anxiety that accompanies agoraphobia can make this form of treatment ineffective unless combined with prescription of a minor tranquilliser.

Hypochondriasis and hysteria

We now enter one of the least well-defined and most contro-versial areas of psychiatry where the patients' production of 'unexplained and ill-defined symptoms is only matched by the

223

psychiatrists propensity for the production of ill-defined diagnostic labels' (Thorley and Stern 1979, p. 231). Hypochondriasis and hysteria have at various times been thought of as different expressions of the same condition with hypochondriasis mainly affecting men and hysteria mainly women. Definitions of hypochondriasis centre around bodily preoccupation, morbid fear of disease and an unshakeable conviction of the presence of disease in spite of reassurance and attempts at persuasion that nothing is wrong. Most hypochondriacs seem to have an underlying psychological problem with depression being probably the most common, and the escape into preoccupation with a physical symptom is thought to be one way of unconsciously alleviating or diverting the emotions from the original troubles. The attention that comes from visits to the doctor, repeated examinations and investigations, and the disproportionate amount of time spent with the patient's troubles may only serve to reinforce the hypochondriacal behaviour and further displace the underlying depression (or whatever) from the surface of the patient's emotional world. Some sort of balance therefore often arises with the continuation of the physical symptoms being necessary to maintain emotional stability. Many hypochondriacs therefore often do not want to be cured of their physical symptoms and repeated visits to one or many doctors becomes a part of their life. Dizziness is one of the many ways in which hypochondriasis can present and the management depends on determining the background disorder that has 'caused' the self-preoccupation to arise. Of course organic disease must be excluded first and this means extensive history-taking, a complete physical examination, and where necessary, appropriate investigations. If it is felt that depression is the underlying cause then appropriate treatment often results in the hypochondriacal symptoms fading away as the depression lifts. However, depression is not always in the background of hypochondriasis and indeed there is some suggestion that in a few patients the symptoms are primary. In all these cases and when there is good evidence that there is no physical disease at work, then formal psychiatric help should be sought. The referring letter should contain the results of all the investigations performed, since for the psychiatrist to repeat them not only increases the cost but also reinforces the hypochondriac's preoccupation with himself.

Hysteria and hysterical personality types as mentioned in Chapter 2 are not different degrees of the same thing. The expression of the hysterical personality is built around the need of the affected individual to appear both to themselves and to others as more than they are and to experience more than they are capable of. This 'is not contrived consciously but reflects the ability of the true hysteric to live wholly in his own drama' (Jaspers 1923). Around this core has arisen a characteristic set of traits that have been described by Chodoff and Lyons in an article well worth reading (Chodoff and Lyons 1958). These traits are:

1. Egotism, vanity and self-indulgence;
2. Exhibitionism, dramatisation and a tendency to tell extravagant and fantastic falsehoods centred about themselves (pseudologia phantastica);
3. Irrational, unchecked and capricious emotionality;
4. Emotional shallowness, fraudulent effect;
5. Lasciviousness, sexualisation, coquetry;
6. Sexual frigidity and fear of mature sexuality;
7. Demanding and dependent behaviour.

This list can of course be interpreted as a warped male view of the female personality and indeed these 'hysterical' traits are found in patients with other psychiatric disorders to the extent that the concept of the hysterical personality type as defined by Chodoff and Lyons becomes difficult to sustain. The core of the hysterical personality — that is, the need to feel and experience more than is actually present and to convince others that it is so — has a reality and is one recognised and disliked by many doctors. The 'exaggeration' of symptoms of dizziness, the inability, for example, to perform a Romberg's test without nearly toppling over in spite of an apparently near normal lifestyle, frequently inhibits proper evaluation and examination. Many will have an underlying problem with balance and are unwittingly driven by their personality to emphasise the symptoms. Their 'gain' by these actions can be interpreted as a reduction in anxiety and an increase in care and attention. Once the doctor has established that nothing is seriously wrong physically, discharging the patient from care may lighten the doctor's load but does little to help the patient, and so psychiatric referral or psychotherapy may be needed if the individual is ever to come to terms with their personality and re-enter 'normality'.

Hysteria which is probably better called a conversion

225

reaction may happen to arise in individuals with a hysterical personality but is not an extension of that personality type. Perhaps hysteria is best thought of as a form of dissociation from unacceptable reality or conflict thereby allowing the individual to cope with the situation (Thorley and Stern 1979, p.217). Hysterical vertigo can thus arise from underlying depression or result from extreme 'stress' with the symptoms and attention received sublimating the underlying problem. As this problem is treated or recedes the hysterical symptoms fade. In many cases of 'hysterical' dizziness however there is an underlying organic disease and Dix (1973) states that 'pure hysterical vertigo is seldom encountered and careful examination nearly always reveals some underlying vestibular abnormality.' Thus, for the patient who has only symptoms of vertigo a rigorous search should be made for disease in the labyrinth and brain before psychiatric referral. Even then the hysterical symptoms may occur before disease is detectable by present-day techniques.

Dizziness frequently forms one of the range of symptoms of a conversion reaction and in this mixed picture may be amenable to psychiatric treatment which resolves the underlying depression or conflict.

18

Management of the Dizzy Patient

If an underlying cause can be found, then in many instances treatment of this alone will result in a cure of the dizziness. The appropriate management of specific conditions or the need for specialist referral has been indicated in the preceding chapters. In many cases however, some remedy for the dizziness will also need to be given whilst the specific treatment is taking effect or whilst natural compensation is occurring. 'Treatment' falls into three categories that can be defined as:

1. enhancing what remains of the system;
2. vestibular exercises in the form of physiotherapy; and
3. medications.

VESTIBULAR ENHANCEMENT

Since the vestibular system functions by integrating the sensory input from several different sources, the diminution or loss of information from one source can, to some extent, be overcome by enhancing or improving the input from what remains. The patient's vision should be the best possible and a visit to the optician for the correct lenses, or to the ophthalmologist for the treatment of cataracts may provide that extra bit of visual input to banish the unsteadiness. The same can be said for the provision of one or two walking sticks to enhance somatosensory input by way of the arms. The patient's shoes should not have thick soft soles as these lessen tactile information from the feet.

227

VESTIBULAR EXERCISES

The vertigo and unsteadiness that come from troubles in the ear, neck or some of the central pathways are characteristically made worse by head movement, so that the patients tend to hold themselves very stiffly, keep their eyes directed straight ahead and to turn with their whole body to look sideways. The problems are worse in the dark and on difficult terrain. Moving about like this is tiring and the fatigue that accompanies the insecurity can push the patient into inactivity and psychological helplessness. The major acute problems often settle spontaneously, or with treatment, but the residual unsteadiness coupled with the lack of confidence can leave the patient 'crippled'.

To overcome some of these problems, a set of exercises was devised by Cooksey (1945) and Cawthorne (1945) with the specific aim of:

1. loosening up the muscles of the neck and shoulders to overcome the protective muscle spasm and tendency to move in one piece;
2. training eye movement to be independent of the head;
3. practising balance under everyday conditions;
4. practising the specific head movement that causes the dizziness to encourage central compensation;
5. getting used to moving about naturally in daylight and in darkness;

and most importantly:

6. encouraging self-confidence in everyday conditions, and assisting psychological adaptation to the residual unsteadiness that in the elderly may never recover completely.

It is very important to explain to the patients in simple enough language what has happened to their balance system, why they feel the way they do, and what the exercises are trying to achieve. They should be told that miraculous, overnight cures are not to be expected and that they must persevere for the outcome is almost certain to be successful. The sooner they can return to normal activities, work or sport, even though it can be difficult early on, the sooner the problems are likely to resolve. The patient should also be told to find the head position and specific movement that causes the most problem and practise making this movement so that the brain can learn to deal with the upset more effectively.

If a relative or friend can help with the exercises and with encouragement then progress is often quicker. Group therapy also has some advantages for beginners in that the sight of improvement in others who are further advanced in treatment is usually encouraging and progress seems to be more rapid.

The exercises are in graded levels and someone still vertiginous and unwell with, say, vestibular neuronitis or following a head injury will need to progress gently through the levels. Another with longstanding problems can progress more quickly although, in general, the order of exercises should not be varied and everyone should start at Level 1.

Level 1: Eye exercises: head kept still

(may be in bed if patient is acutely ill or sitting)
Look up then down, keeping the head still, at first slowly, then quickly. 20 times.
Look from one side to the other, head kept still, slowly then quickly. 20 times.
Focus on a finger held at arm's length then move it about twelve to fifteen inches towards your nose, then away again. 20 times.

Level 2: Head and eye movements

(in bed or sitting)
Bend head forwards then backwards with eyes open, slowly then quickly. 20 times.
Turn head from side to side, slowly then quickly. 20 times.
As the dizziness improves repeat Level 2 with eyes closed.

Level 3: Arm and body movements: sitting

(if previously in bed repeat Levels 1 and 2 sitting)
Shrug shoulders. 20 times.
Circle shoulders. 20 times.
Turn from the waist to the right then the left. 20 times.

Bend forward to pick up an object from the bed, or from the floor if sitting in a chair. Sit up, then bend down to replace the object. Repeat 20 times.

Turn head from side to side, two slow turns then one rapid turn, hold for a few seconds then do three quick turns. As improvement continues repeat with eyes closed.

Level 4: Standing up

Repeat Level 3.

Move from sitting to standing with eyes open. 20 times.

Repeat with eyes closed.

Throw a tennis ball, or the like, from hand to hand, making sure that the ball goes above eye level. 20 times.

Bend forward and pass the ball from hand to hand behind one knee. 20 times.

Repeat with eyes closed.

Change from sitting to standing, turn around once, then sit again. Repeat 10 times.

Level 5: Moving about

Walk across the room, around a chair and then back across the room. After 10 repeats, attempt with the eyes closed.

If in a group or with a friend or relative, practise throwing a large ball back and forth, and then with the patient walking in a circle around the ball thrower.

Step up onto and down from a box or platform. Eyes open first then after 10 repetitions with eyes closed.

Then any game involving stopping or aiming such as bowls or skittles.

A sheet containing an explanation of the reasons for the exercises and clear instructions should be provided if the patient is going to perform them at home with a friend.

DRUG TREATMENT

Although drugs are more commonly the cause of dizziness than an effective treatment for it, there are nevertheless still times when some form of medication needs to be prescribed. There are many problems with deciding what is the best drug to use and this arises because the exact physiology of most vestibular disorders is not really understood and because dizziness tends to resolve spontaneously. This has meant first, that logical or rational therapy cannot be planned and second, that the evaluation of the efficacy of any drug is extremely difficult.

Nevertheless, some drugs have been found to be useful especially in those patients with acute vertigo caused by labyrinthitis, injury or vestibular neuronitis. Three classes of drug are in use; the antihistamines, the phenothiazines and the anticholinergic drug hyoscine. They are listed in Table 18.1.

Unfortunately, there are no proper studies of their usefulness during illness although there are studies of their relative efficiency in motion sickness because of the economic importance of this problem in space flight. Hyoscine (scopolamine) appears to be most effective and prochlorperazine the least, although there are great differences in an individual response, with some doing well with a drug that had no effect on others. Whether these findings can be extrapolated to apply to patients with an acute disease is questionable.

Because of vomiting during the acute severe illness it is sometimes necessary to give the drug intramuscularly or perhaps better by suppository when absorption is rapid. This

Table 18.1: 'Vestibular sedatives'

Class of drug	Drugs	Single dose (mg)	Action (h)	Available
Antihistamines	Cinnarizine	15	4–6	o
	Promethazine		8	
	theoclate	25		o
	Hydrochloride	25–50		o, im, iv
	B Dimenhydrinate	25–50	4–6	o, im, iv, suppos.
	Cyclizine	50	6–8	o, im
	Flunarizine (not in UK)	20	24	o
Phenothiazines	Prochlorperazine	5	4–6	o, im, suppos.
Anticholinergics/ parasympatholytics	Hyoscine hydrobromide	0.3–0.6	1.5–3	o, im (TD not in UK)

Key: o, oral; im, intramuscular; iv, intravenous; TD, transdermal patch; suppos., suppository.

limits the choice a little but as soon as the vomiting has settled an oral agent can be used, and cinnarizine is possibly the most effective since the severity of the drowsiness — which is the disabling side-effect with all these drugs — is relatively low.

Much more common than acute severe vertigo is chronic unsteadiness with the occasional bout of minor vertigo. The first thing to do here is to closely review the various medications that the patient is taking and stop all the minor tranquillisers, sedatives, antidepressants, anti-emetics, vestibular sedatives and vasodilators that have been prescribed, more in desperation than hope of a cure of dizziness. Most of these have side-effects that effect balance and prochlorperazine, acting as a phenothiazine, is particularly good at aggravating postural hypotension and in the long-term causing Parkinsonism, especially in the elderly. The psychotropic drugs — sedatives, antidepressants and tranquillisers — act directly on the central nervous system and probably confuse central vestibular pathways and thereby delay normal compensation.

The next thing to do is to wait for two or three months, getting the patient to start some vestibular exercises in the meanwhile. At the end of this time many will have recovered spontaneously and those that have not can be started on cinnarizine while they continue the exercises.

19

Glossary of Hearing Test Terminology

In the context of the dizzy patient audiometric tests are used to determine whether any associated hearing loss is conductive and caused by problems in the outer and middle ears, or is sensorineural and caused by disease in the cochlea, the cochlear nerve or subsequent neural pathways. If the hearing loss is sensorineural then some of the procedures can help define the location of the lesion as cochlear (sensory) or retrocochlear (neural). The limitations of audiometric tests are that although they can usually indicate that something is wrong, and can often suggest where the problem is, they cannot make a specific diagnosis and therefore can only form part of the framework of investigations.

BASIC AUDIOMETRIC TESTS

Pure tone audiometry

The pure tone audiogram records the quietest sound that an individual can just hear for a range of different tones or frequencies. To test the whole of the auditory pathway in one ear, air-conducted sound produced by some sort of headphone is used. 'Sound' produced by a force transducer (vibrator) placed firmly on the mastoid bone tests the response of the cochlea and subsequent neural pathways. Air-conduction (AC) and bone-conduction (BC) levels are therefore measured and assessment of these two allows the label of conductive or sensorineural to be placed on any hearing loss, provided the tests are performed correctly. The signals presented are usually short bursts of pure tones in the range of 125 to 8000 Hz (cycles

233

per second) for AC and 250 to 4000 Hz for BC. The level of the sound produced by the headphone or vibrator is measured in dB (deci-Bels). The dB scales leave some people a little confused, but they are not too difficult to understand. The scale is based on the ratio of the intensity of the sound in question to the intensity of some arbitrary reference sound. For audiometric purposes the reference sound is the faintest sound that normal young adults can just hear at any specified frequency. Now the range of noise in the environment is so great that using a simple ratio becomes impractical and so the logarithm of the ratio is used to give reasonable numbers. This value is the Bel. Unfortunately the Bel is a bit large for day to day purposes as to express commonly used intensities often involves writing a decimal point, e.g. 6.5 Bels. Therefore a decibel scale is used and, for example, 6.5 B becomes 65 dB.

Thus the value in Bels $= \log_{10} \dfrac{Is}{Ir}$

where

Is = the intensity of the sound in question and
Ir = the intensity of the reference sound,

and the value in dB $= 10 \log_{10} \dfrac{Is}{Ir}$

So far this definition has been derived using sound intensities, but what is more easily measured is the sound pressure level, and this is proportional to the square root of the intensity.

ie.

$\quad P \quad = K\sqrt{I}$

where

$\quad P \quad$ = sound pressure level and
$\quad K \quad$ = a constant.

Thus

$\quad P^2 \quad = K^2 I$

and the dB level using sound pressure levels is

$$dB = 10 \log_{10} \frac{(Ps)^2}{(Pr)^2}$$

with the K values cancelling out.

This is equal to:

$$dB = -20 \log^{10} \frac{Ps}{Pr}$$

At the threshold of hearing the sound pressure is the reference pressure so the dB level is

$$dB = 20 \log_{10} \frac{Pr}{Pr}$$

$$= 20 \log_{10} 1$$

as $\log_{10} 1 = 0$

$$dB = 0$$

The standardised reference pressure is commonly taken at 20 μPa (micro Pascals), so a sound with a pressure level 10 times the reference level will have a dB rating of

$$dB = 20 \log_{10} \frac{200}{20}$$

$$= 20$$

and for a 100-fold increase in the pressure level (i.e. 2000 μPa)

$$dB = 20 \log_{10} \frac{2000}{20}$$

$$= 40$$

If the pressure is one-tenth of the reference level, that is 2μPa then the dB rating is

$$dB = 20 \log_{10} \frac{2}{20}$$

Now $\log_{10} 0.1$ equals minus 1 (-1)

so that $dB = -20$

It is now clear, I hope, that each 20 dB step is a ten-fold increase in sound pressure and if you do the sums slightly differently a 1 dB change is equivalent to a 12 per cent change in the sound pressure level.

Using a sound-level meter to measure traffic noise, industrial noise or even the sound coming out of the hearing test headphones, some reference level, commonly 20 μPa would be used, and the results expressed as dB SPL (sound pressure level). For testing hearing, the reference pressure levels at various audiometric frequencies have been internationally defined so that an individual's threshold at any one frequency can be written as, say, 20 dB HL (hearing level). HL does not mean hearing loss. As with any biological measurement there is a range of normal values, and for the normally hearing population, although the average threshold is 0 dB, the range is from minus 20 dB to plus 20 dB, as some normal people have slightly better hearing, some slightly worse. Thus a hearing level of 20 dB could indicate normal hearing or a loss of 40 dB from a previous threshold of minus 20 dB.

Some more specialised hearing tests are performed with sounds that are louder than the patient's threshold (dB HL), and the difference between this and the level used is called the sensation level (dB SL): so if the threshold is 30 dB HL and the test is performed with a tone of 70 dB SPL, then the tone used is at 40 dB SL.

The symbols to represent air and bone conduction are shown in Figure 19.1. The stapedial reflex threshold will be described in the section on tympanometry.

Audiograms showing typical conductive, sensorineural and mixed losses can be found in Figure 19.2. In general terms a conductive loss with an air-bone gap of around 60 dB is indicative of ossicular discontinuity or of major fixation of the ossicles. A perforation of the drum, or fluid in the middle ear is unlikely to result in a gap of more than 40 dB unless there is another pathology. A sensorineural loss can be high tone, low tone or for all frequencies and, unfortunately, the shape of the audiometric curve is not indicative of the cause. However, noise damage or head injury frequently causes an initial loss at 4 kHz, although as noise-induced hearing loss progresses the damage spreads to involve more frequencies.

One of the problems with testing an ear with poor hearing is that the test sound can frequently be heard in the non-test ear and so give an inaccurate result. If the air-bone gap is more than about 40 dB in one ear then testing air conduction in that ear is likely to give a false result because the sound is heard in the good, non-test ear. The same is true when testing bone conduction on an ear with any hearing loss, as bone-conducted sounds are very easily transmitted through the skull to the other ear. The way out of this problem is to make a masking noise in the

Figure 19.1: The symbols used in British Audiometric procedures and throughout this book.

British Audiometric Symbols

Unmasked bone conduction threshold : △

Right		Left
○	Air conduction threshold	✕
[	Masked bone conduction threshold	]
(	Stapedial reflex threshold	)
Σ	Comfortable loudness level	⅀
L	Uncomfortable loudness level	⅃

non-test ear. The best noise to use is a narrow band of frequencies, centred around the test tone used in the other ear. The masking must neither be too quiet nor too loud to be effective and standardised masking procedures are used to ensure this. Audiograms showing unmasked bone-conduction thresholds are really of no value in assessing the type or degree of a hearing loss and should be ignored.

Speech audiometry

One of the problems with pure tone audiometry is that the procedure does not test for the ability to hear the kinds of

Figure 19.2: Three typical audiograms from patients with hearing loss. **(a)** A pure conductive loss in a patient with otosclerosis. There is in addition a 2 kHz dip in the bone conduction thresholds. This is called a Carhart notch and is typical of stapedial fixation. **(b)** A sensorineural loss — in this case from an elderly man with presbycussis. **(c)** A mixed conductive and sensorineural loss that resulted from a mastoidectomy for extensive cholesteatoma.

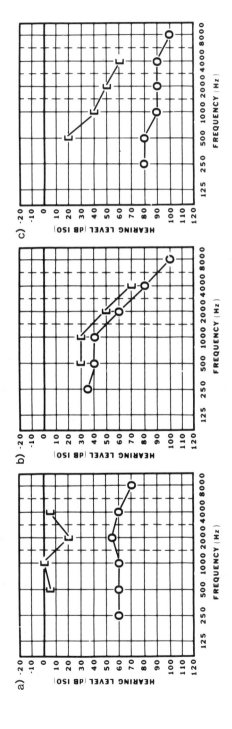

sounds that occur in everyday life, and patients with brainstem or cortical problems may have normal pure tone audiograms but difficulty in hearing or comprehending the spoken word. Speech audiometry therefore uses speech presented either as familiar two-syllable words with equal stress on each syllable — these are 'spondees' and examples are cowboy, blackbird, pen-knife — or as phonetically balanced words. A phoneme is the small identifiable part of a more complex sound, so that the syllable — cat — has three phonemes — k, a and t. Phonetically balanced word lists contain the same proportions of each phoneme — and there are 24 vowel and 20 consonant phonemes in English — as occur in the spoken language. Such word lists are called PB lists. Gaining in popularity are word lists where each phoneme only occurs once (e.g. Boothroyd word lists) or where each word in the list contains two constant and one variable phoneme — pail, fail, sail, tail. The California consonant test is one popular form of this.

Whatever list is used, the essence of the test is to present the word list at one intensity and score the percentage of correct replies. A new list is then presented 10 or 20 dB 'louder' and the new percentage recorded. This is repeated until the plot of percentage response against dB is complete. Figure 19.3 shows a normal speech audiogram. There is a gradual increase in understanding until the 100 per cent comprehension level is reached. The slope will vary depending on the word list used and the presenter's tone of voice.

Figure 19.3: Normal speech audiogram curves for two different forms of word presentation. Spondees are two syllable words with equal stress on each syllable.

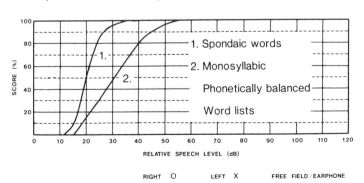

A conductive hearing loss pushes the whole curve to the right, whereas a cochlear lesion results in an additional failure to reach the 100 per cent level. Neural involvement or neural degeneration often causes 'rollover' of the speech audiogram (Figure 19.4) and this result is a relatively good indicator of neural pathology, although it cannot distinguish between pathology in the cochlear nerve and brainstem, nor differentiate between neural loss caused by, for example, an acoustic neuroma, and the degenerative neural loss that eventually results from cochlear damage.

Tympanometry

Although pure tone audiometry is good at indicating the presence and degree of conductive deafness it cannot predict what is likely to be the cause of the particular problem. Direct observation of the ear will show if the canal is occluded, if there is a perforation of the eardrum, and it is usually possible to tell if there is fluid in the middle ear. However, there are other causes of a conductive deafness that cannot be determined by inspection alone and tympanometry can help unravel these.

When a sound enters the ear canal, some of it is absorbed by the tympanic membrane and ossicular chain and enters the

Figure 19.4: Speech audiograms in conductive, cochlear and neural hearing losses. The neural (or retrocochlear) loss is typified by the 'rollover', although this can sometimes be caused by a longstanding cochlear loss with secondary neural degeneration.

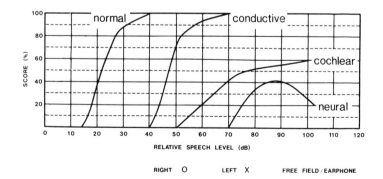

cochlea, whilst the rest is reflected from the eardrum. Under optimum conditions very little bounces back and the acoustic admittance is high. The opposite of admittance is impedance and in the optimum conditions the impedance is therefore low. If the eardrum or ossicular chain is altered then, depending on the condition, more or less sound bounces back and the admittance is changed. This value can be measured but unfortunately single readings — so called static admittance values — do not give much useful information because of the wide range and overlap of values that occur in health and disease. Tympanometry overcomes this problem to some extent by measuring the admittance as the air pressure in the ear canal is varied above and below atmospheric.

An air tight, soft rubber probe is placed into the ear canal to form a seal. The probe contains a small loudspeaker delivering a constant 85 dB SPL, 220 Hz tone, a small microphone and an open duct connected to both a manometer and a pump capable of raising or lowering the pressure in the canal (Figure 19.5).

In the normal ear, the admittance is greatest when there is atmospheric pressure on each side of the drum. As the pressure in the ear canal is raised or lowered the eardrum is distorted and becomes less efficient so that the admittance decreases. This is

Figure 19.5: Diagram of a typical tympanometer. The ear plug contains a small loudspeaker and microphone, and a variable pressure duct. The oscillator delivers a constant background 85 dB 220 Hz sound but in addition is capable of producing tone bursts at different frequences and intensities on top of the background sound.

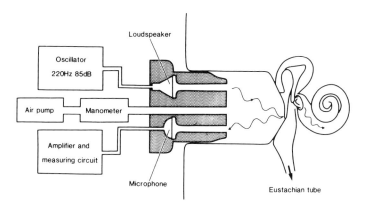

detected by an increase in the sound level detected by the microphone, and is expressed graphically as admittance against ear canal pressure (Figure 19.6).

Fluid in the middle ear, and the associated low pressure that results from Eustachian tube dysfunction (see Chapter 5) decreases the admittance and shifts the peak value to the left, that is, into the low pressure range. When the drum is completely immobile the tympanogram is virtually flat (Figure 19.7). A flat tympanogram can also be caused by a hole in the eardrum or impacted wax but these can be seen by direct observation. If the probe is incorrectly placed in the ear canal so that the tip is lying against the canal wall, the same pattern can also occur but is distinguished by the initial measurement of static admittance (when no pressure is applied) being zero, or very close to zero.

Sometimes a tall, peaked tympanogram is seen and this indicates that part of the middle ear mechanism is hypermobile. It can be a floppy scarred eardrum, or discontinuity of the ossicles. The reverse also occurs to a lesser extent when the ossicles are fixed by, say, otosclerosis, when a low peaked, but normally placed tympanogram is obtained (Figure 19.8).

Figure 19.6: A normal tympanometric curve. The admittance is recorded on the y-axis and the pressure applied to the ear drum on the x-axis. The normal range for the peak of the admittance curve is indicated by the box.

Normal (Type A) Tympanometric Curve

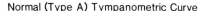
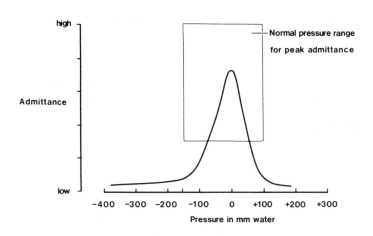

Figure 19.7: Typical tympanometric curves in Eustachian tube dysfunction indicating low middle ear pressures and even immobility of the drum when 'glue' is present.

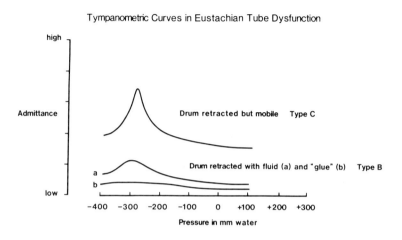

Tympanometric Curves in Eustachian Tube Dysfunction

Figure 19.8: When the middle ear structures are lax, perhaps caused by dislocation of the incudo-stapedial joint or a mobile scar on the ear drum, the tympanogram is tall and peaked. The converse, a normally placed but low-peaked tracing is typical of ossicular fixation.

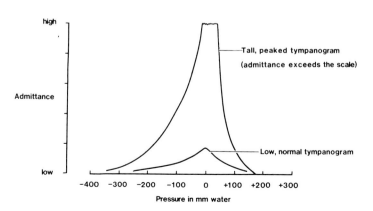

Tympanometric Curves in Laxity and Fixation of Middle Ear Structures

243

Stapedial reflexes

Tympanometry has another useful attribute that arises from its ability to detect movement of the eardrum and changes in the stiffness of the ossicular chain. In response to a loud enough sound the stapedius muscle contracts and pulls the stapes a little so that the ossicular chain is less mobile. This reduces the admittance a little but to an extent that is measurable. The test is usually performed at the pressure that gives optimum admittance, and a loud pure tone is added to the background 220 Hz measuring tone. If the reflex is present the admittance drops and stays low until the loud pure tone is switched off when it returns to its pre-test level (Figure 19.9).

Normally the pure tone needs to be about 70 dB SL to

Figure 19.9: A normal stapedial reflex. When the stimulus is turned on the stapedius contracts and there is a change in the admittance. This change is maintained with little if any decline, whilst the stimulus is present. As soon as the stimulus is turned off the stapes relaxes and the admittance returns to its previous level.

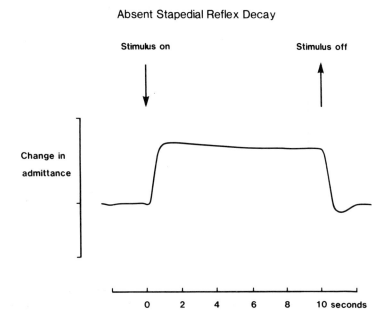

Absent Stapedial Reflex Decay

initiate a reflex so that if there is more than a moderate conductive loss it may not be possible to produce a loud enough sound to activate the reflex. If there is a cochlear loss, the normal 70 dB SL required is greatly reduced and the reflex makes its appearance much closer to the patient's hearing level. This phenomenon is called recruitment, and other tests to establish this feature are described below.

If there is a neural, or more central lesion, the ability to maintain the contraction of the stapes, whilst the loud tone is present, declines, and the reflex decays with time (Figure 19.10). This feature is called 'tone decay' and is another way of separating a retrocochlear from a cochlear lesion, provided the frequency used to perform the test is not 4 kHz or more when some decay occurs in normal individuals.

Figure 19.10: The stapedial reflex is not maintained in this ear and has decayed with time. To be abnormal the reflex admittance must have declined to less than 50 per cent of its initial value but then is a good early indicator of neural (retrocochlear) disease.

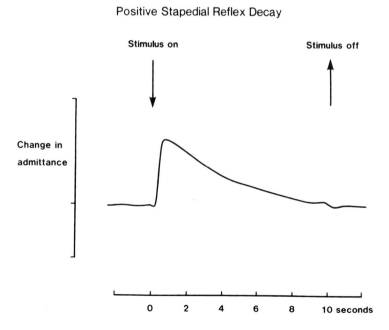

Positive Stapedial Reflex Decay

TESTS TO DETERMINE SITE OF LESION

Recruitment

Recruitment results from cochlear lesions and can be defined as an abnormally large growth in the loudness perceived by the patient as sound intensity (or pressure) increases. The practical expression of this is often seen when talking to older people with presbycussis. When spoken to quietly they fail to hear. They still cannot hear when the voice is raised a little and then a little more, until they suddenly say 'Don't shout — I'm not deaf'. For an explanation of the mechanism of recruitment Pickles' excellent book *Physiology of Hearing* (1982) should be consulted. There are many ways of detecting recruitment. The stapedial reflexes are a good and simple method but two other procedures are in common use.

Alternate binaural loudness balance (ABLB)

The ABLB was first described by Fowler in 1928 and the test consists of the patient determining the level at which pure tones seem equally loud in both ears. This test is only useful when there is one relatively normal ear and one ear with some degree of sensorineural loss. After a pure tone audiogram has been performed, a test tone at 20 dB SL for the good ear is presented to that ear for a moment. The tester then presents a brief tone of the same frequency at 20 dB SL to the bad ear and the patient is asked if it is louder or quieter than that heard in the good ear. Depending on his response the second tone is made louder or quieter and again compared with the 20 dB SL in the good ear. The procedure is repeated until the two sounds appear equally loud and the dB levels are recorded. The tone in the good ear is increased by 10 or 20 dB SPL and the procedure repeated until four or five different sound levels have been tested. These results can be plotted as shown in Figure 19.11 which shows both a normal result and one with recruitment. For completeness different frequencies can be tested and then it is sometimes simpler to present the results as a 'laddergram' (Figure 19.12).

Short increment sensitive index (SISI)

This test consists of superimposing short-lived increments of 1 dB on top of a sustained tone of 20 dB SL at each frequency

Figure 19.11: Fowler's alternate binaural loudness balance. The normal result in a patient without recruitment as well as conductive or neural lesion is on the left. A 'recruiting' ear with an abnormally large growth in loudness with increasing sound intensity is shown on the right. The square boxes indicate the level of the sounds in each ear that appear equally loud.

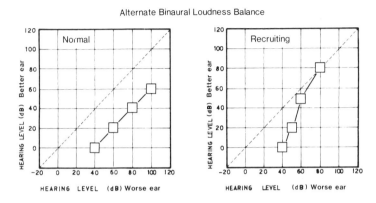

Alternate Binaural Loudness Balance

tested. The patient is asked to push a signal button whenever any increment is heard whilst listening to the sustained tone for two minutes. During the last twenty 1 dB increments each lasting 200 ms are presented and can be interspersed with 5 dB increments. Only the positive responses to the 1 dB increments are scored and the percentage recognised calculated.

In general, normal people and those with conductive and neural losses yield low scores below 30 per cent, whilst cochlear losses show high or very high scores. Presbycussis is unpredictable, presumably because the nature of the loss is both cochlear and neural.

Tone decay

The inability to continue hearing a continuous pure tone presented a little above the threshold for pure tone represents the phenomenon of tone decay and when present is a good but not absolute indicator of neural involvement. There are many ways of attempting to elicit tone decay but the various procedures fall into two basic types; threshold and suprathreshold testing.

247

Figure 19.12: An alternative way of presenting the results of recruitment testing allowing several different test frequencies to be shown at once. At any one frequency the levels which appear equally loud are joined by a heavy line. With recruitment the 'steps on the ladder' stop being parallel and bunch up on the bad side.

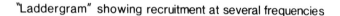

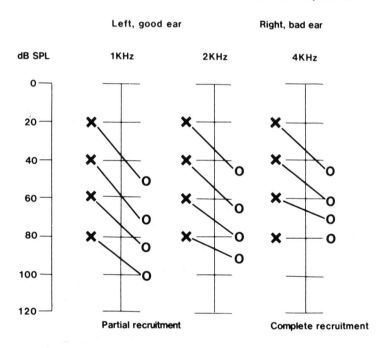

"Laddergram" showing recruitment at several frequencies

Threshold tone decay

Depending on the procedure a pure tone is presented to the test ear at 5 or 20 dB SL and either the time in seconds (up to 60) that the tone is heard is recorded, or the increase in dB required to maintain audibility for one minute noted. Complete tone decay occurs when no intensity can be heard for the full minute. When 25 dB SL has to be used to maintain audibility then this is considered to be positive for a neural lesion. The diagnostic significance is increased if there is complete decay, if there is abnormal decay at several frequencies, or if the decay occurs rapidly with each increase in intensity.

Suprathreshold adaptation tests

These tests were developed because it was felt that tone decay could be detected earlier by using high intensity rather than near threshold pure tone levels. The patient separately listens to tones at 500, 1,000 and 2,000 Hz, presented at 110 dB SPL for one minute, with the non-test ear appropriately masked. Any inability to hear the test sound for the full minute is taken as a positive sign of neural involvement, and again, the value of this sign is enhanced if there are abnormal findings at several frequencies, and if the decay occurs rapidly.

ADVANCED AUDIOMETRIC TESTS

Bekesy audiometry

Apart from winning one Nobel prize, Georg von Bekesy also found time to develop a form of automated audiometric testing that now carries his name. Various modifications of the original design have been made since, but the essence of the test machine is a sound production device that slowly and continuously increases the frequency of the test tone. On top of this is a separate control affecting the intensity of the sound that is worked by the patient. When the control button is pushed the sound intensity decreases and the patient is asked to keep the button pressed while he continues to hear the sound. When the sound is no longer heard, the button is released and the intensity increases again. There is normally an 8 to 12 dB difference in the level at which the sound is heard to go off and the level at which it is heard again as the intensity increases. This on/off effect is recorded on an X-Y plotter as the machine sweeps continuously through the frequencies (Figure 19.13). The usefulness of this form of audiometry has been enhanced by adding another run through the frequencies but this time using pulsed tones of 200 ms on and 200 ms off. In the normal the pulsed and continuous tracings overlap and this is called a Type I Bekesy audiogram. Other types are found in disease and are listed in Table 19.1. Figure 19.14 shows a result typical of Type V or non-organic hearing loss found in a patient seeking compensation.

Table 19.1: Bekesy audiometry results

Type		Condition
I	Continuous and pulsed tracings overlap throughout the frequency range	Normal Conductive Rarely cochlear
II	Above 1,000 Hz the continuous tracing drops below the pulsed tracing but by less than 20 dB	Cochlear
III	Continuous tracing drops below pulsed tracing at low frequencies, and the gap increases so that by 1,000 Hz the continuous tone cannot be heard at all	Retrocochlear
IV	Constant difference between the two tracings at all frequencies with the continuous tracing up to 20 dB below the pulsed one	Retrocochlear rarely cochlear
V	Marked difference across the frequency range with the pulsed tracing below the continuous tracing — the opposite of Type IV	Non-organic Malingering

Electric response audiometry (ERA)

When a short-lived sound enters the cochlea, some of the sensory cells are activated and the corresponding fibres of the acoustic nerve are stimulated. A short volley of neural impulses therefore passes along the nerve to the cochlear nuclei in the brainstem, and subsequently through a number of other nuclei before reaching the auditory cortex. This defined sequence of electrical activity should therefore be measurable, rather like the electrocardiogram, but the random background electrical noise from muscles, other nerves and the brain, makes picking out this very small auditory signal like trying to find the proverbial needle in the haystack. Fortunately, the signal from the auditory pathway is time-locked, that is, it occurs with monotonous regularity after each sound stimulus. Thus, if the stimulus is repeated at fixed intervals, and the electrical responses recorded for a short while after each stimulus are added together, the background noise will eventually cancel itself out as it is more or less random. The auditory signal will remain intact and will be amplified by the number of repetitions of the signal. With the advent of more sophisticated electronic gadgetry such a procedure is possible and averaging computers are routinely used to record time-locked signals lost in a background of random electrical noise.

Different parts of the auditory pathway can be investigated

Figure 19.13: A Bekesy audiogram using the continuous tone only. An interrupted tone is also used but in the type I audiogram overlays the continuous tone and so has been omitted here for clarity. Various combinations exist and are detailed in Table 19.1.

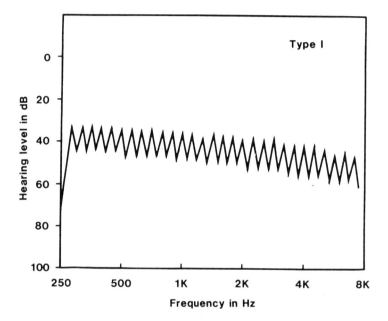

Bekesy Audiometry: Continuous Tone Only

by altering the length of time for which the signal is followed. A short time 'window' reveals early events in the cochlea and auditory nerve whilst a long window can show the signal being received in the cerebral cortex.

Electrocochleography (ECochG)

This procedure records the response from the cochlea and the initial activity of the acoustic nerve. These both occur within about 10 ms of the stimulus, and a typical normal tracing in response to a loud click stimulus is shown in Figure 19.15. As the intensity of the click is reduced, the whole nerve action potential becomes small and the delay in its appearance increases so that the threshold of hearing can be fairly accurately estimated by the disappearance of the waveform.

Figure 19.14: A Bekesy audiogram in a patient with a non-organic hearing loss. The man was involved in litigation over possible noise-induced deafness and although he did have some sensorineural loss it was nowhere near as much as was suggested by his pure tone audiograms and this typical type V Bekesy tracing. The solid lines indicate the continuous tone and the dashed lines the pulsed tones.

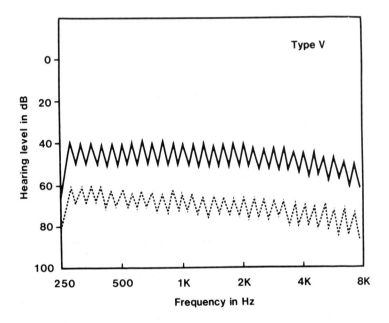

Bekesy Audiometry: Continuous and Pulsed Tones

Different cochlear pathologies alter the shape of the action potential and summating potential and these changes can be helpful diagnostic features.

Brainstem electrical responses (BER)

These are recorded when the analysis time is increased to 20 ms. Several waves are constantly found and are taken to indicate the signal reaching or passing through various parts of the brainstem pathway. Unfortunately, there is still some confusion about naming the various waves and indeed about which is up and which is down. Nevertheless the responses can help in assessing the hearing levels, since pure tones can be used as the

Figure 19.15: The normal electrocochleogram in response to a high intensity click stimulus.

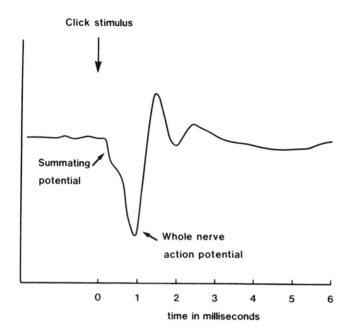

Normal Electrocochleogram at High Intensity

stimulus, and the technique is especially useful in babies as it is non-invasive. Loss or delay of the wave form pattern can also help to site disease and has been useful in detecting small acoustic neuromas, and suggesting brainstem involvement by multiple sclerosis, tumours and even the effects of decompression sickness in deep-sea divers. Finally, the absence of brainstem reflexes in the unconscious patient seems to indicate irreversible brainstem death and the procedure will therefore probably become a useful aid in this difficult area of medicine.

The middle latency responses

These are recorded from 10 to 60 ms and indicate the signal reaching the thalamus and primary auditory cortex. Although theoretically useful the test has not yet become a standard or standardised procedure.

The cortical responses

The cortical responses to sound form part of the electroencephalogram (EEG) and as such were some of the first changes detectable in the days before averaging computers were available. Now that the EEG can be electronically removed the cortical responses have become a useful indicator of an intact auditory pathway. The major responses occur with a delay of about 100 ms, last for about another 100 ms and can be used to determine the threshold of hearing. The results are not quite as sensitive as a conventional pure tone audiogram, but an audiogram can be produced by using different pure tones as the stimulus, and the procedure is particularly useful in children and babies.

The beauty of ERA is that the patient under test need not make a subjective response such as pushing a button. The term objective audiometry is therefore then applied although this is not quite precise as the test still depends upon the observer deciding whether a wiggle in the tracing is a response or not. A good beginners' book on ERA is by Gibson (1978).

BEST TEST COMBINATIONS

No single test can infallibly distinguish cochlear from retrocochlear lesion as each will give some false positive and some false negative results. Thus a combination of tests to sort out the retrocochlear lesion is needed. This test battery should be quick and easy to perform, inexpensive and applicable to most patients. A reasonable combination that optimises the diagnosis is:

1. Stapedial reflex threshold and decay;
2. A tone decay test;
3. A speech audiogram to detect 'rollover'.

The strong suggestion of a retrocochlear lesion on these three tests can be enhanced by finding a Type III or IV Bekesy audiogram and almost certainly confirmed by finding appropriate changes in the brainstem electrical responses.

References

Adler, F.H. (1941) Occular vertigo. *Trans. Am. Acad. Ophthal. Otolaryngol.*, 27-31

Aschan, G. (1958) Different types of alcohol nystagmus. *Acta Otol. Suppl.*, *140*, 69-78

Aschan, G., Bergstedt, M. and Stahle, J. (1956) Nystagmography. *Acta Otol. Suppl.*, *129*, 54-8

Aschoff, J.C., Conrad, B. and Kornhuber, H.H. (1974) Acquired pendular nystagmus and oscillopsia in MS. *J. Neurol. Neurosurg. Psychiat.*, *37*, 570-7

Balkany, T.J. and Dans, P.E. (1978) Reversible sudden deafness in early acquired syphilis. *Arch. Otolaryngol.*, *104*, 66-8

Baraka, M.E. (1984) Rate of progression of hearing loss in Paget's disease. *J. Laryngol. Otol.*, *98*, 573-5

Bender, M.B. (1965) Oscillopsia. *Arch. Neurol.*, *13*, 204-13

Bickerstaff, E.R. (1961) Basilar artery migraine. *Lancet, i*, 15-17

Biemond, A. and Dejong, J.M.R.V. (1969) On cervical nystagmus and related disorders. *Brain*, *92*, 437-58

Brain, R. and Norris, F.H. (1965) *The remote effects of cancer on the nervous system*, Grune and Stratton, New York

Brain, W.R. and Wilkinson, M. (1965) Subacute cerebellar degeneration in patients with carcinoma. In W.R. Brain and F. Norris (eds), *The remote effects of cancer on the nervous system*, Chapter 3, Grune and Stratton, New York

Bretlau, P., Causse, J., Causse, J.B., Hansen, H.J., Johnsen, N.J. and Salomon, G. (1985) Otospongiosis and sodium fluoride. *Ann. Otol. Rhinol. Laryngol.*, *94*, 103-7

British Medical Journal (1982) Alcohol Problems. British Medical Publications, England

Causse, J., Shambaugh, G.E. Jr, Causse, J.B. and Bretlau, P. (1980) Enzymology of otospongious and NaF therapy. *Am. J. Otol, 1*, 206-14

Cawthorne, T.E. (1945) Vestibular injuries. *Proc. Roy. Soc. Med.*, *39*, 270-3

Chodoff, D. and Lyons, H. (1958) Hysteria, the hysterical personality and hysterical conversion. *Am. J. Psychiat.*, *114*, 734-40

Cody, D.T. and Baker, L.H. (1978) Otosclerosis: vestibular symptoms and sensorineural hearing loss. *Ann. Otol.*, *87*, 778-96

Coles, R.R.A., and Knight, J.J. (1961) Aural and audiometric survey of qualified divers and submarine escape training instructors. *MRC Report RNP, 61*, 1011

Cooksey, F.S. (1945) Rehabilitation in vestibular injuries. *Proc. Roy. Soc. Med.*, *39*, 273-5

de Groot, J.A.M., Huizing, E.H., Damsma, H., Zonneveld, F.W. and Van Waes, P.F.G.M. (1985) Labyrinthine otosclerosis studied with a new computed tomography technique. *Ann. Otol. Rhinol. Laryngol.*, *94*, 223-5

255

de Jong, P.T.V.M., de Jong, J.M.B.V., Cohen, B. and Jongkees, L.B.W. (1977) Ataxia and nystagmus induced by injection of local anaesthesia in the neck. *Ann. Neurol., 1,* 240-6

de Lignieres, B., Vincens, M., Mauvais-Jarvis, P., Mas, J.L., Touboul, D.J. and Bousser, M.G. (1986) Prevention of menstrual migraine by percutaneous oestradiol. *Br. Med. J., 293,* 1540

Dix, M.R. (1973) Vertigo, *Practitioner, 211,* 295-303

Dix, M.R. and Hood, J.D. (1969) Observations upon the nervous mechanism of vestibular habituation. *Acta Otol., 67,* 310-81

Dohlman, G.F. (1981) Critical review of the concept of cupular function. *Acta Otolaryngol.* Suppl., *376,* 1-30

Dunlop, E.M.C. (1972) Persistence of treponemes after treatment. *Br. Med. J., 2,* 577-80

Edwards, C.H. (1973) *Neurology of ear nose and throat disease.* Butterworths, London

Ellis, A.E. (1958) *The rack.* Heinemann, London, Reprinted by Penguin, Harmondsworth

Farmer, J. (1977) Diving injuries to the inner ear. *Ann. Otol., 86* (Suppl. 36), 1-20

Fitzgerald, G. and Hallpike, C.S. (1942) Studies in human vestibular function. I. Observations on directional preponderance (nystagmus bereitschaft) of caloric nystagmus resulting from cerebral lesions. *Brain, 65,* 115-37

Forssmann, B. (1964) A study of congenital nystagmus. *Acta Otolaryngol., 57,* 427-49

Fowler, E.P. (1928) Marked deafened areas in normal ears. *Arch. Otolaryngol., 8,* 151-5

Fowler, E.P. (1950) The recruitment of loudness phenomenon. *Laryngoscope, 60,* 680-95

Fregly, A.R. (1974) Vestibular ataxia and its measurement in man. In H.H. Kornhuber (ed.), *Handbook of sensory physiology,* vol. IV pt. 2, Springer-Verlag, New York, pp. 321-60

Fukuda, T. (1959) The stepping test. *Acta Otol., 50,* 95-108

Gacek, R.R. (1983) Cupulolithiasis and posterior ampullary nerve transection. *Ann. Otol. Rhinol. Laryngol. Suppl., 112,* 25-30

Gibson, W.P.R. (1978) *Essentials of clinical electric response audiometry.* Churchill Livingstone: Edinburgh, London

Gibson, W.P.R., Prasher, D.K. and Kilkenny, G.P. (1983) The diagnostic significance of transtympanic electro cochleography in Ménière's disease. *Ann. Otol. Rhinol. Laryngol., 92,* 155-9

Greven, A.J. and Oosterveld, W.J. (1975) The contralateral ear in Ménière's disease. *Arch Otolaryngol., 101,* 608-12

Griffiths, O. (1979) Incidence of ENT problems in general practice. *J. Roy. Soc. Med., 72,* 740-2

Hart, C.W. (1984) Caloric tests. *Otolaryngol. Head Neck Surg., 92,* 662-70

Hinchcliffe, R. (1961) Prevalence of the commoner ear, nose and throat conditions in the adult rural population of Great Britain: a study by direction examination of two random samples. *Br. J. Prevent. Soc. Med., 15,* 128-39

Hood, J.D. and Korres, S. (1979) Vestibular suppression in peripheral and central disorders. *Brain*, *102*, 785-804

Jaspers, K. (1923) *General psychopathology* (Trans. by J. Hoenig and M.W. Hamilton), University Press, Manchester

Karmody, C.S. and Schuknecht, H.F. (1966) Deafness in congenital syphilis. *Arch. Otolaryngol.*, *83*, 44-53

Knox, J.M., Musher, D. and Guzick, N.P. (1976) The pathogenesis of syphilis and related treponematoses. In R.C. Johnson (ed.), *The biology of parasitic spirochetes*, Academic Press, New York

Langton-Hewer, R. and Wade, D.T. (1984) Management of patients with stroke. *Prescribers J.*, *24*, 66-70

Lawton-Smith, J. (1969) *Spirochetes in late seronegative syphilis, penicillin notwithstanding.* C.C. Thomas, Springfield, CI

Lopez Ibor, J.J. (1972) Masked depressions. *Br. J. Psychiat.*, *120*, 245-58

Lundquist, P.G., Rask-Andersen, H., Galey, F.R. and Bagger-Sjöbäck, D. (1984) Ultrastructural morphology of the endolymphatic duct and sac. In I. Friedmann and J. Ballantyne (eds), *Ultrastructural atlas of the inner ear*, Butterworths, London

Marks, I.M. (1969) *Fears and phobias.* Heinemann, London

Matthews, W.B. (1970) *Practical neurology*, 2nd edn. Blackwell, Oxford, p. 69

Mayfield, D., McLeod, G. and Hall, P. (1974) The CAGE questionnaire: validation of a new alcoholism screening instrument. *Am. J. Psychiat.*, *131*, 1121-3

McNulty, J.S. and Fassett, R.L. (1981) Syphilis: an otolaryngologic perspective. *Laryngoscope*, *91*, 889-905

Morgagni, J.B. (1769) *The seats and causes of disease investigated by anatomy in five books.* Translated by B. Alexander, London 1769

Morrison, A.W. (1975) *Management of sensorineural deafness.* Butterworths, London

Morrison, A.W. (1984) Ménière's disease. In M.R. Dix and J.D. Hood (eds), *Vertigo*, John Wiley, Chichester, pp. 133-52

Nightingale, S. (1985) Management of migraine. *Prescribers J.*, *25*, 129-34

Orford, J. (1977) Impact of alcoholism on family and home. In G. Edwards and M. Grant (eds), *Alcoholism; New knowledge and new responses*, Croom Helm, London

Pickles, J.O. (1982) *An introduction to the physiology of hearing.* Academic Press, London

Rogers, J.H. (1980) Romberg and his test. *J. Laryngol. Otol.*, *94*, 1401-4

Royal College of Psychiatrists (1979) *Report of the Special Committee on Alcohol and Alcoholism.* Tavistock, London

Rudge, P. (1983) *Clinical neuro-otology.* Churchill Livingstone, London

Sacks, O. (1985) *The man who mistook his wife for a hat.* Gerald Duckworth, London

Sade, J. (1979) *Secretory otitis media and its sequelae.* Churchill Livingstone, New York, p. 246

Shambaugh, G.E. and Holderman, J.W. (1926) The occurrence of otosclerosis in the aetiology of progressive deafness. *Arch. Otolaryngol.*, *4*, 127-36

Slack, J. (1983) The use of lipid lowering drugs. *Prescribers J.*, *23*, 134-9

Slater, E. (1965) Diagnosis of 'hysteria'. *Br. Med. J.*, *i*, 1395-9

Somerville, B.W. (1975) Estrogen withdrawal migraine. *Neurology, 25*, 239-44

Stahle, J., Stahle, C. and Arenberg, I.K. (1978) Incidence of Ménière's disease. *Arch. Otolaryngol.*, *104*, 99-102

Stephens, S.D.G. (1975) Personality tests in Ménière's disorder. *J. Laryngol. Otol.*, *89*, 479-90

Stokes, W. (1846) Observations on some cases of a permanently low pulse. *Dublin Quart. J. Med Sci.*, *II*, 73

Teasdale, G. and Jennet, B. (1974) Assessment of coma and impaired consciousness. A practical scale. *Lancet, ii*, 81-4

Thomsen, J., Bretlau, D., Tos, M. and Johnsen, N.H. (1981) Placebo effect in surgery for Ménière's disease. *Arch. Otolaryngol.*, *107*, 271-7

Thorley, A. and Stern, R. (1979) Neurosis and personality disorder. In P. Hill, R. Murray and A. Thorley (eds), *Essentials of postgraduate psychiatry*, Academic Press, London, pp. 179-246

Trimble, M.R. (1981) *Neuropsychiatry.* Wiley, Chichester

Tumarkin, A. (1936) The otolith catastrophe: a new syndrome. *Br. Med. J.*, *2*, 175-7

Vercoe, G.S. (1976) The effect of early syphilis on the inner ear and auditory nerves. *J. Laryngol. Otol.*, *90*, 853-61

Walker, G.S., Evanson, J.M., Canty, P.D. and Gill, N.W. (1979) Effect of calcitonin on deafness due to Paget's disease of the skull. *Br. Med. J.*, *2*, 364-5

Watanabe, I. (1980) Ménière's disease with special emphasis on epidemiology diagnosis and prognosis. *ORL, 42*, 20-45

Wilmot, T.J. (1979) Ménière's disorder: a review. *Clin. Otol.*, *4*, 131-43

Wilmot, T.J. and Menon, G. (1976) Betahistine in Ménière's disease. *J. Laryngol. Otol.*, *90*, 833-40

Worth, C.T. and Hussein, S.M.A. (1985) Peripheral neuropathy due to long term ingestion of allopurinol. *Br. Med. J.*, *291*, 1688

Wu, A., Chanarin, I. and Levi, A.J. (1974) Macrocytosis of chronic alcoholism. *Lancet, i*, 829-30

Index